CANCER AND INFERTILITY

A Story of Hope

J. RICHARD SMITH

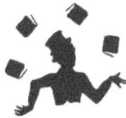

MENSCH PUBLISHING

Mensch Publishing
51 Northchurch Road,
London N1 4EE, United Kingdom

First published in Great Britain in 2023

A catalogue record for this book is available
from the British Library

ISBN:
978-1-912914-50-0 (paperback)
978-1-912914-51-7 (ebook)

Typeset by Van-garde Imagery, Inc., • van-garde.com

Contents

Dedication

This book is dedicated to: Professor Alan and Mrs Andrea Richardson, Rev Gary Bradley, Mr Robert Chandler, Professor Hani and Mrs Diana Gabra, Ms Catrina Donegan, Ms Yeng Poon, Fr Anthony Speakman, my four children, Cameron, Victoria, Madeleine and Lara, and finally last but by no means least my sister and mother, Miss Alison and Mrs Diana Smith; without these people there would be no book. They all know the individual roles they have played over the last few years.

Confidentiality

Patient confidentiality is a time-honoured principle of medical ethics. The patients referred to in this book have given permission for their medical histories to be published. Only names and other identifying details have been altered in order to protect their privacy. Their stories are true and inspiring.

The Derivation of Gynaecological Words

Gynaecology is unusual amongst the medical specialities in that most organs have two names; one Greek derived, the other Latin. Thus hysteros, Greek for womb, is uterus in Latin; Colpos, Greek for a blind ending sac, is vagina in Latin. This follows the same pattern with oophoros from Greek, meaning egg-bearing and ovarium (plural ovaria) or ovary from the Latin; trachelos, the Greek for neck, is the equivalent of cervix, or the 'neck' of the womb. Finally, to break all the rules, there is the Fallopian tube, named after an Italian anatomist, Gabriello Fallopio. Removal of the Fallopian tube is salpingectomy, again derived from the Greek. As you may have noted, if we refer to the organ it is in its Latin form, but if a procedure is to be performed we go to the Greek version e.g. to remove the uterus is a hysterectomy.

Raison D'etre

Every account in this book has been written with patients in mind, every account in this book has been told to my patients, every account in this book appears to have been appreciated by my patients as relating to their healthcare. The mission of this book is to give help and hope to women with cancer and / or infertility.

This book is about hope—hope of a cure, hope of living well with a bad diagnosis, hope of having a baby and, if this proves impossible, the hope of good strategies to live well with the issues that these things create. The vast majority of women and men will go to enormous lengths to achieve long-term remission of their cancer in the hope of cure, but the woman who has cancer and no children will often be quite prepared to risk her life in pursuit of a baby.

This book is about a philosophy of caring in medicine. To state the obvious, care should be centred on the patient and their wishes. Can we always give the patient what they want? No, but we sure can try our best to reach this goal.

No matter how bad the situation may appear, there are ways to make it positive. If you are a woman with cancer or you are infertile that is serious, put the two together and it may feel insurmountable but there are strategies to create hope and relief. Your doctor should never give up and never stop trying to alleviate your suffering.

Every week for more than thirty years, I have sat down in my clinics and seen a sequence of women who are frightened and anxious. Their immediate anxiety stems from simply being in the clinic and having to talk about intimate things with somebody who, at that initial consultation, is a complete stranger. They may have family or friends who have met me before but it is still scary. Some women may have relatively minor problems in the bigger picture, but every one of them has waited anything from days, if cancer is suspected, to weeks or even months if non-cancer problems are the issue: that twenty to forty-five minute appointment is incredibly important for each woman.

If I am going to play it right by every patient, the consultation has to be of the same quality at the beginning, middle and end of the day; this is every doctor's role. It is absolutely not for me to judge the importance of the patient's problem, it is my role to deal with that problem to the best of my ability. Many years ago, I complained to a colleague that the wound in my stomach created by a surgeon the previous day during a 'minor' operation was sore. He replied "the definition of a minor operation is one you are not having yourself." Too true. If you are the patient, your problem is paramount. In any consultation, the woman and I have to get on the same team very quickly if we are going to have success.

My specialist areas within gynaecology are the fields of cancer management and gynaecological surgery, with a particular interest in fertility-preserving surgery as well as surgery designed to improve fertility. I also have had a long-standing interest in infection and immunity. This combination of specialist areas, I believe, encourages holistic thinking.

When a new patient, walks through my door, with a cancer or with infertility or a combination of the two, my earnest hope is that we can assist with both; that her cancer will be cured and she will go on to have a baby. If for any reason we are not successful, these women will need support and assistance to deal with this loss.

The press and the public perception of cancer is always of kill or cure, but this is rarely the case. The majority of gynaecological patients with cancer are cured and the remainder can live for many years with their disease. For those patients who desire to retain fertility, their risks may be increased by their choices which is why it is crucial that their decisions be informed. For those who lose their uterus as a result of cancer treatment, or those who have been born without a uterus, comes the concept of acquiring a new uterus through transplantation. Uterine transplantation has the potential to allow these women to have a baby, and to carry that baby.

Throughout most of our lives we all desire to be whole people, in body, mind and spirit. Disease upsets this equilibrium on all three levels. High quality medicine should strive for restoration.

Golden Rules

The golden rules are designed to guide doctors and patients in the multiplicity of situations they find themselves in across medical care. The Golden Rules are a framework for doctor and patient to work around. I will regularly say to patients "we have a golden rule here" and then illustrate it with the accounts you will find in this book. For some patients this is about cancer care, for others it is about infertility and for some they apply to both, or indeed maybe general to all of medicine.

I have always regarded doctors and patients as being on the same team, no them and us or us and them, which is why these are everybody's golden rules. If you are in the hands of lawyers somebody is going to win and somebody lose, in the hands of doctors everybody is trying to win for you.

Rule 1. Never give up – the story of fertility-sparing surgery and uterine transplantation (cancer care and infertility)

Rule 2 Never say never (cancer care)

Rule 3. Be flexible – adapt to situations as they develop and do not presume to sit in moral judgement (general).

Rule 4. Always tell the truth. "How long have I got, doctor?" – take great care with prognostication (cancer care).

Rule 5. Hit them hard and hit them fast (cancer care).

Rule 6. Never say "There is nothing more we can do" There always is, do not presume to know the patient's desires (cancer care).

Rule 7. If you are the patient, don't lie to your relatives; if you are the relatives don't lie to the patient (cancer care and general).

Rule 8. Understanding personal humility: Doctors might be better doctors if they were patients themselves (general).

Rule 9. Don't frighten the patient. Healthcare professionals need to look the part and engage (general).

Rule 10. A cup half empty can become a cup half full (cancer care and general).

Rule 11. Walk the walk, swim the swim, chant the chant (general).

Rule 12. Fertility, sex and orgasms are life essentials (infertility and general).

Introduction

In 2008 I was walking at the south end of the Isle of Bute when my hospital pager went off. They are now a thing of the past but the rule was—if you can you must always answer. Pagers, ironically, were more efficient at tracking you down, no matter where you were, no matter how remote your location. Garroch Head on Bute sure is remote—four miles of no roads, only sheep tracks and the West Island Way.

There was always a frisson of irritation when the pager went off. One dutifully rang the switchboard, usually after a muttered curse word. This particular afternoon, the switchboard at Charing Cross hospital told me they had a patient who wished to speak to me. That was not the normal deal and my irritation increased. Back then, this involved writing the number down on a piece of paper or the palm of one's hand. Woe betide you if you had forgotten to put a pen in your pocket. I duly phoned the number given and a woman answered.

"Is that you, Mr Smith?"

"Yes, who am I speaking to?" I asked, growing more curious. She gave me her name and the penny dropped, all irritation disappearing in an instant.

"I wanted you to know that I am lying in a hospital bed right now and my new-born baby is beside me."

Every baby is a gift - that goes without saying - but this baby was a very special gift indeed. The mother had recently undergone fertility-sparing surgery for a placental site tumour. This rare and aggressive cancer would normally be managed by hysterectomy but, thanks to the development of a new surgical procedure by our team, we had managed to remove the tumour keeping the womb intact. This woman's success was built upon an evolution of thinking and had been a brave decision on her part. She had been prepared to increase her own risks in the face of an aggressive cancer to be able to have a baby.

The operation is called a Modified Strassman Procedure. This was the first baby ever born in the world to a woman who had undergone such an operation. A determined patient and surgeon, some out-of-the-box thinking and a degree of good luck can sometimes deliver amazing results.

Rule 1.

Never give up —
the story of Fertility-Sparing Surgery
and Womb Transplant UK

A Scottish friend said to me a while ago, "Gee Richard, you have been talking about this operation for a very long time. Is it not about time you actually did it?" A bit harsh, but so true. It's been a long path which started in 1996. I had just been involved with the invention of a procedure to allow young women with cervical cancer to retain their fertility. This operation is called an Abdominal Radical Trachelectomy, and is now performed worldwide to the betterment of many thousands of women. During this procedure, the womb is outside the abdomen attached to the patient via the ovarian blood vessels only. The cervical cancer is then removed and the uterus stitched back onto the vagina. It's almost a transplant.

The concept of trachelectomy came from French surgeon, the late Daniel Dargent, who pioneered vaginal trachelectomy whereby the cervical cancer was removed via the vagina, leaving the body of the uterus intact thus allowing the woman to have a baby. This was, and still is, technically challenging. In 1995 an American surgeon, Giuseppe Del Priore, and I had the good fortune to be at a conference in New Orleans where we heard Dargent present his new operation. We turned to each other and discussed whether or not the procedure could be done more easily via an abdominal approach. Opening the abdomen had been the standard approach to removing cervical cancers for decades. We returned to New York and, via the anatomy department of Bellevue Hospital, performed an initial abdominal radical trachelectomy in a human cadaver: it worked! I returned to London and obtained ethics approval to perform an abdominal trachelectomy en route to a radical hysterectomy in a woman with a cervical cancer: again, it worked. We then collaborated with Lazlo Ungar in Budapest and the operation of abdominal radical trachelectomy was born.

I knew it was firmly established when I was having breakfast with my two older children in a New York diner. On the radio playing in the background came an advert from Memorial Sloane Kettering cancer centre saying "If you are a young woman with cervix cancer, you don't need to lose your fertility, come to Memorial Sloane Kettering for an abdominal trachelectomy." I turned to my children and said "That's Dad, Giuseppe and Lazlo's op."

Following that preliminary procedure, where we performed the trachelectomy but then proceeded on to a hysterectomy, I sat down in the pub with my great friend and '"big brother', Sam Abdalla. As you will discover, he taught me how to hypnotise people. For many years, Sam ran Lister Fertility, London, the UK's biggest IVF unit. It was 1995 and we were in the Rising Sun pub behind the Lister and I was excitedly describing our first trachelectomy case and then we moved to uterine transplantation— were there women who might benefit from such a procedure? Sam had some stats, there were approximately 50,000 women in the UK with absolute uterine factor infertility, in other words they had either been born without a uterus or their uterus had been removed for one reason or another. Of these women of course, many had no desire for a baby or already had one. However, he also knew that 100 to 200 women per year went down the route of surrogacy because they had no uterus. Sam knew there were many women at Queen Charlotte's with Mayer Rokitansky Küster Hauser Syndrome (MRKH) who had been born without a uterus. They did, however, have ovaries and a vagina. I had no idea then that there were around 6000 women in the UK in this position. One in 5000 women born in the UK has this condition. I realized I had been thinking like a cancer surgeon—we were taking wombs out that women really didn't want to lose, could we help them to retain them by trachelectomy or maybe give them a new womb further down the line? It now transpires that the majority of women seeking a womb transplant have MRKH syndrome and are not cancer patients. Less than 20% of the women who have approached us have had cancer. However, this does not detract from the linkage between fertility preservation and restoration, all designed to allow women to carry their own baby.

The full story of Womb Transplant UK is told in another of my books, *Womb Transplant UK: an Epic Journey* (World Scientific).

It's interesting because out of these many thousands of women we have been approached by over 500 directly and, after email contact, we came down to just over a hundred serious contenders. On further enquiry, this came to a little over 50 women. Womb Transplant UK's remit is to fund the women and the NHS for ten transplants where the donor is deceased—a heart beating brain dead cadaver (DBD). These are donors who, for one reason or another, are brain dead but on a ventilator in intensive care. Their relatives are approached at what is an exceedingly difficult time to ask if organs can be retrieved and, if so, which. This DBD process forms the foundation of all liver, pancreas, heart and lung transplant programmes worldwide. We also know that across the South East of England, with a population of approximately 20 million people, this will render between 10 to 20 suitable uteruses per year. My guess looking to the future is that there will be two UK centres for DBD, one in the north of England in Manchester, Liverpool, Leeds or Newcastle, that arc of cities having a similar population conurbation. We also planned under the auspices of the charity to perform five transplants from living donors (LD), where the donor of the uterus is either the mother or sister of the recipient.

LD transplants may become more available across multiple units, although it is difficult to see where the funding will come from in a cash strapped health service. We have applied to NHS England to set up a National Uterine Transplant Centre based between Oxford and Imperial College to open in 2027 to allow NHS funded DBD cases at the rate of 10 per annum. This has been signed off by the Secretary of State for Health, the centre being contingent on the success of the above 10 DBD cases.

In the Rising Sun, we talked long that evening over the technical challenges and an idea was born. The challenges were around the technicality of removing the womb with its supplying blood vessels and then finding out where to connect them. There was also a worry about whether a blood vessel which had been cut and stitched back together would work during pregnancy. To explain, if you are unfortunate enough to have your hand taken off in an accident the blood vessels supplying your hand are 2-3 mm in diameter and they are always that size. A womb, however, is different. A non- pregnant normal uterus is the size of pear, the woman about to deliver a baby has a womb the size of a watermelon. The pear-sized womb has blood vessels of 2-3mm diameter, the watermelon sized uterus has blood vessels which have expanded to 1 cm in diameter in order to supply the growing uterus and baby contained within it. In addition to this, the pear-sized uterus sits in the pelvis, not even palpable in the abdomen until a woman is 12 weeks pregnant. By the time of delivery the top of the uterus is under the ribs. The vessels have to grow not just in diameter but also grow longer. Normal uterine vessels don't just look like a tube, they look like the coiled cable in an old-fashioned land line telephone; the cable connecting the phone to the hand-held part. I've always found this amazing.

We also talked about the possible success rate of such a procedure. Sam was in the IVF field from very early on and I remember the first year of IVF in Glasgow. £250,000 worth of drugs were administered in the programme to the women of Glasgow resulting in one baby. That, at the time, was the experience everywhere. Contrast now with the huge success rates of IVF. For womb transplants, what would be regarded as good enough by way of success at the start, and what would be the consequences for the patient and the team in the event of failure?

There were also the worries about infection risk. Other organs like kidneys, heart, lungs are all removed from a sterile body cavity in the donor and inserted into a sterile body cavity in the recipient. Not so with the uterus, since the vagina always naturally contains bacteria. We speculated that evening if the uterus would be better put into the recipient with no connection to the vagina, but then would come the issue of where menstrual blood would go, or whether one would need to give drugs to stop menstruation. These bacteria in the vagina might infect the new uterus and the transplant would fail. Then there was the worry about immunosuppressive drugs that all transplant patients have to take, to stop them rejecting their new organ. Would they harm the baby? We know from the tens of thousands of kidney transplant women who have had babies that the increased risk of miscarriage is minimal and there is no increase in congenital abnormalities in their babies. Beyond this, it is well recognised that long-term immunosuppressive therapy can lead to cancer and increased risks of infection in the patients taking these drugs. In the transplant world, most organs that are transplanted are considered to be vital. In other words, you can't survive without a functioning heart, lungs and liver. Without a kidney, you must have dialysis to survive. For decades, because of all these risks, there was no consideration of transplanting non-vital organs. However, with ever more sophisticated drugs for immunosuppression and improved monitoring, non-vital organs came on the agenda about 20 years ago. The non-vital organs considered were hands, limbs, faces and then wombs entered the picture. The upside of a non-vital organ transplant is that if anything goes wrong with the new organ the patient can survive if it is removed—not the case with the heart. With the uterus, it was immediately obvious that the goal of the new womb would be to allow a woman to have a baby but once she had delivered one or maybe two babies, it would then be removed and the woman could stop her potentially dangerous immunosuppression. It is interesting to note that the risk of cancer rises with the greater number of years of taking the drugs, so in the women who might have a womb transplant they would maybe take the drugs for 2 to 4 years.

In fact, moving forward to 2023, our protocols have patients on immunosuppressive drugs from the time of their transplant for 6 months of monitoring, then they have an embryo put into the uterus. 9 months later, the baby is delivered by Caesarean section and then 6 months later they have a hysterectomy or move forward to have another baby and repeat the process. It has even been mooted that this uterus, when it comes out, could be used again, quite a thought.

Having moved forwards to 2023, it is noteworthy that having now met many women requesting a womb transplant there is much more to this than just having a baby. Many women who have no uterus do not feel whole. Part of the desire for a uterus is to fulfil that deep inner need. When we started the trachelectomy work we originally thought that women would have hysterectomies after they had completed their families to minimise their risk of cancer recurrence. This has not happened at all. The cure rates proved to be similar to hysterectomy so to remove the uterus would be to increase the risks by going through more surgery. However, I have only had one trachelectomy patient ever request a hysterectomy. Looking way into the future, with tissue engineered wombs, there will be no need for the immunosuppressive drugs and I will bet there will be no women wanting their new uterus removed; I might be wrong.

Returning to that evening in the Rising Sun, Sam and I emerged; I realised that many of the technical issues we had identified could never be addressed without doing some preliminary work in an animal based laboratory. We went through the appropriate training and exams to allow us to do this. We were incredibly fortunate to meet Professor David Noakes, at the Royal Veterinary College (RVC), London who played a huge role over many years. What we discovered over that time led directly to the story of the woman described in the introduction to this book— the world's first woman to have a baby following a fertility-sparing procedure for her rare cancer. It also allowed us to realise that we could divide vessels, stitch them back together and there was no hour glass effect as we had worried about. Unfortunately, we then went on to discover that to use these small uterine arteries in a transplant didn't work and the uterus shrunk over time, not a good result. This, following advice from transplant surgeon Professor Nadey Hakim, led to the use of larger vessels to allow the blood supply to function properly. This is the technique which has now been applied in uterine transplantation worldwide. New techniques for assessing transplanted organs via multi-spectral imaging have also been developed as a result of this research.

In addition, the operation described in the introduction—the Modified Strassman Procedure—was developed on the back of these ideas. We realised that we could temporarily block off the blood supply to the uterus thus allowing us to open it, even cut the body of the uterus in two with ultrasound during the operation to identify the tumour, then cut it out with a margin, stitch the uterus back together, allow the blood to flow back in and we had a normally functioning uterus allowing the patient to have a baby. We have used the same technique to dilate the cervix from the inside out where it proved impossible vaginally, leading to embryo transfer and successful pregnancy.

As we touch on animal based work this is probably a good time to discuss ethics! The rules around animal based work are, quite rightly, extremely strict and I can reassure you that the standards of care for the animals are of the highest level. All our work was Home Office licensed and inspected and went through the RVC ethics committee. No work was ever performed that was not going to have a direct outcome for humans at a future date; in addition, no work was carried out in an animal model if it could be performed ethically in a human setting. Once the Swedish team had their successful human transplant, which I talk about later, all our animal uterine transplant work ceased forthwith. I make this important point because when you publish scientific work it usually goes into print anything up to two years after the work was performed.

In the early days of this project, many ethical issues were debated about whether it was right or wrong to even consider transplanting wombs in women. The usual way this gets thought through is via what are called The Four Pillars of medical ethics. These are: first, do no harm (*Primum non nocere*). Womb transplant fails on this one, but so does much of modern medicine.

Second, do good (beneficence), Womb transplant gets a tick here. Transplanting wombs is about the begetting of babies and that constitutes one of the strongest aspects of human flourishing, something that medicine is meant to be all about.

Thirdly, autonomy: this is respect for the aware patient who understands the risks and benefits of a proposed procedure and duly consents in full knowledge of these facts; womb transplantation scores very highly on this pillar.

The fourth pillar is justice, a concept familiar to all of us, and again womb transplantation gets a tick here. In the early days we had two senior ethics advisers who both believed that to consider transplanting wombs was entirely acceptable, in fact ethically superior to surrogacy.

I was a bit shocked in 2016 to receive an invitation to a two-day meeting solely on the subject of the ethics of uterine transplantation. I had not thought there was enough to talk about; I was wrong. This took place at the University of Lancaster and a fascinating meeting it was. Much of the discussion took place around the ethics of transgender patients. In the UK, under The Equality Act 2010, male to female transgender patients have the same rights as any other woman, assuming technical feasibility. But when it comes to technical feasibility there are many problems. These include the narrow triangular shape of the male pelvis instead of the wide cylindrical shape of a woman's pelvis. There is no intention of any women with transplanted wombs delivering normally. They are all delivered by Caesarean section. It is rather the difficulties of inserting the uterus into a narrow space and allowing the vessels to be connected. Also, we know that the womb transplants performed where there was not a natural vagina have not fared well, with multiple miscarriages. For this reason, in our protocols if you are a woman without a 'normal' vagina you are not allowed to be considered for the procedure. I would say that while it is ethically appropriate to consider uterine transplantation in the transgender setting, it will prove technically highly challenging, and is a good way off.

Up until 2014 when the Swedes had their great success, transplanting the uterus in nine women, I had personally received a hard time at multiple scientific meetings, in fact usually getting an easier ride from the press. The whole project seemed to create controversy and stimulate highly polarised responses from friends and colleagues.

Over the years, there have been many splurges of publicity where there is a media feeding frenzy lasting 24 hours and it then dissipates. Womb Transplant UK has been so fortunate to have had the support of Neil Huband of Priority Counsel to keep us out of trouble, this he has so generously done *pro bono* to help us. It's worth pointing out that including the research fellows, who were actually paid to be Resident Medical Officers and not to undertake research, no member of the extended team has ever received a penny of recompense excepting basic expenses. This amounts to such generosity on the part of over twenty-five senior medics and scientists over decades.

To illustrate the strong feelings engendered, after one of these media hypes, I turned up at work. I stepped into the lift and a breast surgeon stepped in. She immediately congratulated me on my research. I stepped out three floors up and a nurse congratulated me. I then walked around the corner past another surgical colleague who said "Richard, your research is a load of shit!" In addition to this, at multiple meetings, doctors would question the sanity of any woman thinking about undergoing this procedure. These factors and an inability to obtain mainstream research grants lead Srdjan Saso and me to perform surveys of staff, both medical and nursing, and also to gauge acceptability in potential patients. In depth, psychological studies were set up as well. These all showed in the main a lot of support across the board and that the potential patients were sane and fit to plead. This is borne out by hard data from Dr Stina Jarvholm, the psychologist with the Swedish Uterine Transplant group lead by Professor Mats Brannstrom. The first nine women to undergo this procedure have been extensively studied by Dr Jarvholm and found to be very level, aware of the risks and benefits, as were the nine living donors. Even in the two women where the procedure failed and the uterus had to be removed, they expressed no regret that they had undergone the procedure and in fact one would like to try again.

Returning to matters financial, one of the great difficulties we have had throughout the decades has been lack of financial support. Our research has led to over ninety peer-reviewed publications but we have never received a mainstream grant. We have been fortunate to receive support from a number of private charities and have been overwhelmed by the generosity of the public; people holding events, doing charity walks and runs etc. This issue was ironically highlighted in a recent exchange of letters in the *Daily Mail*. The first letter stated that this type of work was a waste of NHS resources; the irony is we have never used any and the charity's stated goal is to fund the first fifteen transplants at no cost to the health service. Happily, another member of the public wrote back to say they knew our team and that much good had come from our research for NHS patients at no cost to the NHS. You might imagine, and you would be right, that there is a little plea here to your generosity. The website will be included at the end of this chapter.

Returning to criticism of the project, I myself have not been without the odd wobble as to whether we really were doing the right thing. The first international meeting of the various groups took place in Gothenburg in 2007. There were delegates from the UK, USA, Colombia and of course our Swedish hosts. I have to confess to returning to London thinking maybe we were not doing the right thing by trying to progress this. I was lucky that evening that my friend Catrina Donegan came for dinner. She is a senior nurse who happens to have had a liver transplant herself and was on the UK Womb Transplant Advisory Board. I leant across the table. "Catrina, you've had a transplant, you take the medications every day, if you had been born with no womb, would you have a uterine transplant?" I think if she had said "No" I might have given up. Happily, "Yes, absolutely, I would, for sure," came the response. That made me feel much better. Within a day or two I had met another woman requesting the procedure. As always, when you hear the stories of these women, it fires the desire to try and do something, it's always heart rending. I once had a patient who told me her story.

"I went through my early teenage years and, unlike my friends, my periods never arrived. I was sixteen and my mother and I thought I should get some advice. We went to the doctor who referred us to the local hospital where we saw a gynaecologist. Blood tests were ordered and a scan. It was at the scan. They could see my ovaries, but no womb, it wasn't there. I always wanted children.

"Of course, it's all so personal and private and you can't talk to anybody about it, it becomes a big family secret. What do I tell my boyfriend? When do I tell my boyfriend? Will he leave me when he knows?"

Until the possibility of womb transplantation, the only fertility options were adoption or surrogacy, the latter not an option if you are a Muslim or an Orthodox Jew.

The juxtaposition of dinner with Catrina and seeing this new patient convinced me that I should keep going. In addition, the many spin offs over the years have kept us all going and continue to do so. Transplant surgeons do much work on organs when they are out of the body with no blood supply, but this is a whole new concept for gynaecological surgeons. It is, however, on the horizon that certain procedures on the uterus could be undertaken with the uterus outside the body, still attached by two vessels only, these are temporarily blocked and abnormalities removed from the uterus with minimal blood loss.

Also within the group of women who have approached us there are some who have a normal womb, but no lining to their womb. The endometrium is missing. This is called Asherman's syndrome. We currently have a Fellow in tissue engineering looking to grow endometrium from stem cells to address this issue without the need for either a uterine transplant or taking any immunosuppressive drugs. A further possibility we have investigated is to transplant only the endometrium itself from live donors. This would be a much smaller retrieval procedure from the donor, a simple hysterectomy only with no requirement to take any surrounding blood vessels. The endometrium would be cut out of the uterus that had been removed and then the recipi-

ent's uterus opened having blocked off the blood supply temporarily, and stitched in. Our original work in this area produced
variable results but in our last project combining a new process
called PRP (protein rich plasma) with the transplant we appear
to have achieved normal endometrium and we are about to apply
for Ethics Committee approval to move this technology into the
human setting.

One of the things which has amazed all of us over the last
four years is the hundreds of women who have approached us
looking to donate their uterus, entirely altruistically. Because
of the nature of the retrieval we have politely declined, this may
change. I suspect, however, that the majority of living donors will
continue to be mothers and sisters.

In 2014, I was invited to Bristol to give a lecture on uterine transplantation. I have given this talk many times over the years, with
the content continuously being updated and revised. I enjoy lecturing but always feel nervous beforehand—public speaking and
surgery share one thing for sure, you are only as good as your last
lecture/operation. A lack of nerves or preparation can prove
disastrous. Years ago, I had a lecture on HIV which took me all
round the world; I gave it over 60 times. Usually it was well reviewed by the audience and went well. There were, however, two
memorable occasions where it completely bombed, a very uncom-
fortable feeling when nobody even greets you or talks to you after
you finish—coffee on your own, everybody else standing chatting. Worse, when you reflect back later, you can't see what's gone

wrong and therefore can't assuage any anxieties before you give it again. Personally, I think some audiences just take against you, if they do you're stuffed. Anyway, back to Bristol, where the talk in fact went exceedingly well. I returned to London by train and phoned young Saso, who was my fellow at the time, to tell him about the talk; this not something I would normally do. My reason was that for the first time ever the audience were on side with the concept of uterine transplantation. There was no criticism at all, just encouragement. This was a first in 18 years. I said to Saso that I thought our time had finally almost arrived. We had a good chat and then rang off. A few minutes later my phone rang, I was not in the quiet carriage, and I answered it. The news had just broken about the success of the Swedish trial. Mats Brannstrom and colleagues had delivered a woman with a transplanted womb at 32 weeks gestation of a live healthy baby. Wow, what a result. Until it had been done, nobody knew whether it would work. The Rubicon had been crossed. It had shown great bravery on the part of the patient, her family and the surgical team. They had also done incredibly well to protect the woman from the world's media. This was a momentous afternoon. We were intending to apply for ethics approval ourselves around that time. I had been reading Saso's thesis which was in preparation and of course Mats's work was much referenced. What I'd spotted was that he had hit seventy peer reviewed publications in 2012 and felt it was the right time to go for ethics approval in Sweden. We had hit the seventy publications in late 2014, much due to the 'peer reviewed paper publishing factory' that was and is Saso, and were applying in

2015. The Swedes really deserved to be first, at that point we were trailing along about two years behind them.

The Swedish approach of planning to do ten cases had proved a masterstroke. They in fact performed nine cases; two required the uterus to be removed within the first three months, one because of infection, the other because the blood vessels got clotted up. Of the remaining seven women, six have gone on to have one or two children. One, who did not have her own natural vagina, sadly had a number of miscarriages. This is an astoundingly successful set of results for a first trial. Of the seven women who retained their new uterus there was a 100% pregnancy rate and an 85% baby rate, quite amazing. Interestingly there was also a very low rate of miscarriage, perhaps as a result of the immunosuppressive drugs, although that is speculation. Compare this with the success of IVF in the early days.

All these cases utilised living donors and the retrieval procedures took up to 13 hours. It was this length of retrieval procedure which made us decide that in the UK we would go down the deceased, brain dead (DBD) donor route. In surgery, there is a risk of deep venous thrombosis (DVT), this is clot formation in the large veins in the leg and pelvis; it's a particular risk with pelvic surgery and the risk rises the longer the operation. Procedures over six hours make this particularly risky. Sometimes a piece can break off the clot landing in the lung, this is called a pulmonary embolism and can result in death. It is important to say that I am in no way implying that it was unethical to do what was done but just not right for us in the UK. Over the ensuing years, over ninety cases have been performed worldwide, with many babies born. Most of the cases have retrieved wombs from living donors and the majority of babies born have been born to living donors. There are two amazing statistics: if you have a uterine transplant you have a 20% chance it will not work and the uterus will have to be removed in the first few weeks after the operation, however if you have a period after the transplant, and 80% do, virtually everybody goes on to have a baby.

So, what happened to the UK effort? We managed to get ethics approval in 2015, following a very helpful conference with Mats and the Swedish group. They very generously shared all their protocols, which much helped our cause.

Just after this I had the great privilege to be a co-organiser of a conference in Leipzig, Germany, the home of Bach and also the great German surgeon Michael Hockel. Michael is not only a great surgeon but a startlingly innovative surgical scientist. He has formulated the theories about why cancers only cross certain barriers late on in their development, which is down to where the tissue derived from during development as an embryo. A really good example of this is in cervical cancer, which starts in the cervix and then tends to spread to the upper vagina or the tissue either side of the uterus or to lymph nodes. Why does it only very late on spread to the bladder and bowel, both of which directly lie beside these tumours? The bladder, the bowel and the cervix develop from different tissue when the foetus is about 8 weeks old; this creates a 'natural' barrier. Professor Hockel has developed a surgical approach based on these theories. My co-organiser during this meeting was

Stephen Kennedy, Professor of Obstetrics and Gynaecology at the University of Oxford. Stephen is a truly wonderful man. He and I have lectured together many times. His research is on how babies grow in the womb and thereafter. This has been a huge international undertaking led by him which has shown that it is'all down to the nutrition of the mother, none of it is racially pre-determined as was previously thought. Every time I hear him lecture, I just think, how great is that? Ironically he seems to feel the same way about my talk. After we had both spoken we agreed to meet for a drink before the conference dinner. Stephen suggested that perhaps a way to break certain political impasses, in which we were enmeshed at the time, would be to share the project with the University of Oxford. I duly went up to Oxford and a new collaboration was born. We found new and wonderful colleagues in the Churchill Hospital Department of Transplantation Surgery, with transplant surgeons Miss Isabel Quiroga, Professors Peter Friend and Rutger Ploeg and Mr Venkatesha Udupa. Ironically, I was in Oxford a while back at the same surgical group conference as in Leipzig. We were staying in the Cotswold Lodge Hotel opposite the restaurant we met in three years earlier and during this conference the legal documents between Imperial College and the University of Oxford were finally signed off.

In the December of 2015 our team went to Oxford where we met and started to work with Miss Isabel Quiroga, Consultant in Transplantation Surgery specialising in renal and pancreatic transplants. Thus started an essential collaboration leading to our eventual success. We were certified by NHS Blood and

Transplantation (NHS BT) as official organ retrievers. From then, until the summer of 2016, we performed a number of dry runs and practise retrievals. Throughout that year we attended multiple meetings where we presented our project to all of the interested parties. These included the transplant surgeons, the intensive care anaesthetists, the specialist nurses for organ donation and the transplant physicians. This resulted in our getting approval from the Research, Innovation and Novel Technologies Advisory Group (RINTAG) and the Human Tissue Authority (HTA) in December 2016. In January 2017, the NHS BT senior management committee gave us provisional approval. I am aware this will seem to be huge amount of bureaucracy, but at the end of the day it is vitally important that our team do nothing to besmirch the reputation of transplant surgery in the UK or in any way damage the already existing difficulties within the DBD programme of obtaining enough organs for vital organ transplants. We, as a team, have always been aware that we must do nothing to upset that process. Utterly integral to this process has been Research Fellow Mr Benjamin Jones, a great doctor and a very skilful negotiator and facilitator. Ben is now the Post Doc and continues to produce academic papers at a prodigious rate. He, Saso, Isabel Quiroga, and I, have presented multiple times to all the various stakeholder groups. We have had some hairy times, nerve wracking times and much fun.

In March 2017, Ben and I had the privilege of presenting at the British Transplant Society meeting in Harrogate and were truly welcomed as part of that community, a really important step for us. For me there was a great opportunity to meet two of the great doyens of transplantation, Sir Roy Calne, who for years I believed was mentioned in Billy Joel's song, 'We didn't start the Fire.' My sister informs me I have misheard and the song but I will never hear it any other way.

The other person was Professor Roger Williams CBE, with whom I had a personal connection, albeit distant. I walked along with him between sessions at the conference and was able to re-count a referral our team had made to him in 1983 when I was a houseman in the Southern General Hospital; there's a lot about those days in this book. There was a man I admitted as an emergency who had sadly decided he wished to kill himself and had swallowed 200 paracetamol tablets and then sat around at home for two whole days. He had then decided that he had made a mistake and brought himself to the hospital where I admitted him. His liver function tests were disastrous and death sadly looked inevitable. The Registrar on call with me was Dr Bob Kilpatrick (sadly deceased), a great character and an excellent doctor. In the ward office, I said, "Bob, I was listening to Radio 4 a few days ago and heard this Professor Roger Williams from King's College Hospital, London being interviewed. He talked about a new thing called charcoal haemoperfusion, the equivalent for the liver of dialysing a kidney. Maybe we could refer this poor guy there?" Bob looked at me and without hesitation picked up the phone and called switchboard.

Professor Williams agreed to take the case and suggested Bob transfer the patient to Glasgow Airport by ambulance, fly him to London and he would arrange a chopper to bring the patient into Kings. This duly happened. Bob and I were feeling very proud, we reckoned we had scooped the award for best referral of the year!

The following morning we did, however, find ourselves in hot water. Our boss Dr Adams (known behind his back as Jock) appeared on the ward for his round. He always started by reading the nursing notes before he heard any of our presentations. As this man had gone to London we would not have presented him anyway; he was after all no longer our patient. Of course, he looked up from the nursing ledger.

"Did you fellows transfer a patient to Kings?"

"Eh, yes."

"How did he get there?"

"Eh, we sent him in an ambulance to Glasgow Airport, plane to London, chopper into Kings."

The look on Jock's face was a picture. "Did you guys not think to phone the consultant on call—me—and at least discuss it before you blew thousands of pounds of Glasgow Health Board money?"

Well the look on our faces said it all. Bob said, "Eh, we should have thought of that."

At this point a glimmer of a smile appeared on Jock's face. "There are a lot of rules about ordering up helicopters and putting sick patients on airplanes, it seems we have broken all of them. Having said that you gave the guy a chance. Please don't repeat this stunt."

It should be said that Jock himself flew planes and was a fellow of the Glasgow, Edinburgh and London Royal Colleges of Physicians and rumour went he had flown himself between Glasgow and London when taking those exams, I guess in the 1940s or early 50s. We had the right boss to survive this communication breakdown. Now for the good news, the patient survived, and in fact he returned to our ward in Glasgow a few days later hale and hearty to complete his recovery; what a great result. I took great pleasure, 34 years later, in meeting Professor Williams, the man himself, and recounting the story.

In addition, there was another happy piece of chance at the conference. I had the privilege to give the penultimate talk, and I then walked out into the foyer. Those Yorkshire boys who were running the conference centre wanted us all out and had opened the front doors of the building, a freezing cold gale was blowing through. There were, however, free sandwiches, and as a good Scots boy I felt duty bound to have my free lunch. I zipped and buttoned up my coat and sat down at the one free table to partake of my sandwich. The next thing, a very charming man also in a suit and coat buttoned up comes over. "Do you mind if I sit at your table, all the others are taken?" I of course replied, "You are most welcome." He sat down and introduced himself as the CEO of Organox.

"I enjoyed your talk very much." I thanked him. "Do you know about our device?"

"Oh, I sure do, I went on a course about your device, so interested in it are we, but we can't afford it!"

He retorted with "You can now, it would really help you."

Now the device in question is a piece of machinery, about the size of a Renault Twingo car. It is a warm perfusion device designed for livers. To explain, when organs are removed from brain dead donors they are chilled to preserve them but there is a limited time that the organ is viable for; this creates a great urgency to implant the retrieved organ into the recipient woman. For wombs, ideally the timing is under 12 hours, but up to 24 hours is acceptable, each organ varies, for livers it's 12 hours. This has the capacity to create much disruption when our rota goes live, one week on, one week off. If we could use a warm perfusion device, perhaps we could retrieve on a Wednesday and implant on a Saturday thus minimising disruption every which way. A new collaboration was happily formed over that cool lunch and we began working with their scientists.

Over the next months, the various legal processes and contracts were signed. All through this time our sole goal was to pursue the 10 DBD cases. Isabel Quiroga and colleagues in Oxford put in a power of work to make this happen. Then came the second Gothenburg conference in October 2017, this proved a real game changer.

It was slightly sad for our team since we had fallen behind internationally with many countries moving forwards and performing mostly live donor transplants. In our defence, we were trying to set up a sustainable programme of DBD transplants, not to just do a few cases and we had decided not to do live donor transplants. Imagine then, on the second day of the conference,

Liza Johannesson, who used to work with Mats in Gothenburg and then went on to Dallas, presented new data on a new method of retrieving the uterus from live donors. I listened in amazement. The retrieval involved taking out the uterus and upper vagina, as expected, but the vessels used, instead of the big pelvic arteries and veins as in all the previous live donor cases, had now been changed to the big arteries but the small ovarian veins as the drainage vessels. This was astounding on many levels, so much so that after Liza gave her presentation I ran down the stairs at the back to grab her at coffee time and check I had understood correctly. Firstly, this new approach had cut the retrieval time for 10 to 13 hours described earlier to 4 to 6 hours; you remember all that stuff earlier about deep venous thrombosis and pulmonary embolism—problem massively reduced! In addition, the risk of injuring the ureter, the tube between the kidney and the bladder, was also much reduced. The Swedish group had one injury to the ureter in the original nine cases. Of course, the most shocking thing of all to me personally was that retrieval had become the abdominal trachelectomy procedure we originally described in 1995, which had led on to all this work on uterine transplantation. It was staring us in the face but we had failed to see it was the solution to living donor retrieval. A journalist asked me what I had thought at this moment. "I knew I was a complete a... hole." She kindly described this as my *Eureka* moment, but it wasn't, Liza had the Eureka moment. From that moment, it became obvious that the science had changed and we needed to do live donors as well as our DBD programme. In addition, ironically, the live donor procedure is now so well established with such success as to no longer be considered pure research. This was the point that our team changed our goal from 10 DBD research cases alone to doing 10 DBD research cases and five live donor cases. The reason DBD remains research is that while there are a number of successful transplants currently there are only a few babies born after this procedure.

In January 2020, our team went on call for deceased donor transplants and by the end of February we had been called six times, three times the donor was unsuitable and three times the families refused to let any organs be retrieved. Our first living donor case was booked for mid-March. Then Covid-19 arrived and of course everything went on hold. Two and a half years later, with much politics and effort from Isabel, Ben, our new Fellow Dr Saal Vali and myself, all permissions were back in place. Our study, collaborative between Imperial College, London and the University Of Oxford, was back on track. We were on call for deceased donor transplants.

In late 2022 the team, led by Isabel Quiroga, and me successfully retrieved a uterus and its surrounding vessels. That night I discovered a new word, 'explant', that is the retrieval. We arrived in Oxford to perform the implant, the explant and the implant together making the transplant. We met our recipient patient and her partner on the ward and expected to be sending for her within the hour. This was an emotional moment for all of us, the couple themselves and Ben, Saal and me on this pre op ward round. None of us could quite believe we were there.

Isabel was already in theatre starting the back table work. The graft looked perfect but when we did the cannulation, whereby we put tubes into each of the vessels which are intended to be used for joining up (anastomosis) we found the left internal iliac artery and its uterine artery were perfect, the two ovarian veins were perfect as were the two internal iliac veins leading to the uterine veins. Then to our horror we discovered that the right uterine artery was completely blocked with atheroma; no amount of effort relieved this situation and the decision was made to stop the procedure. Very sadly we went to the ward to see the patient and her partner; this was a very distressing meeting which Isabel handled with great sensitivity, skill and compassion. This patient went back on our list for when the next suitable organ became available.

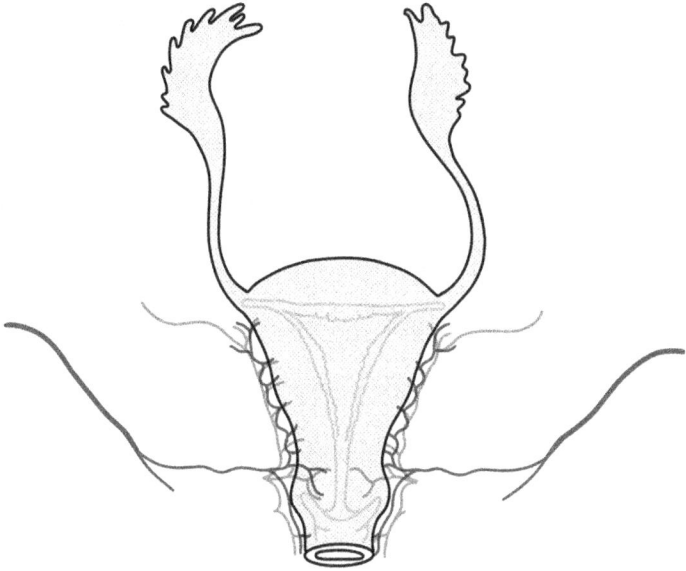

Fig 1: Deceased donor uterus graft with vessels

At the feedback meeting later in the week we were asked "Who held the scissors?" I laughed and said "Both Isabel and I held the scissors. We have done a lot of operating together in the laboratory and have very complementary skills." In truth we are very lucky as a surgical duo that we can operate backwards and forwards without ego; I am the lead for the retrievals (explant) and Isabel the lead for the implantation (implant). What was also clear that night was that we gynaecologists were in a different arena from our own and without Isabel I would have found the going in general very tough and the retrieval impossible. We discovered that our surgical skill sets were different. I, as a cancer surgeon, expect to remove a diseased organ with a margin of 1 cm normal tissue around it and I seal vessels using various devices, the organ removed goes to pathology. Isabel, as a transplant surgeon, removes viable normal organs for implantation into another patient, no margin of normal tissue is required but rather an organ in good condition with its supplying vessels intact and undamaged. This requires great care tying small vessels and much less use of sealing devices. So as the retrieval progressed I would say "seal?" Isabel would say "tie" or "yes," she also often using the sealing device where appropriate. So much was learned and gained. We had done very well with our first explant, and the explant itself was a huge success in surgical terms, although very difficult for our recipient.

We returned to Oxford staying in the Cotswold Lodge Hotel again. I had dinner at Gees restaurant opposite, where I had been "interviewed" all those years before to bring the project to Oxford. I met early that evening with Isabel, and later Ben and Saal arrived at Gees. The following morning, in early February, we left the hotel at 6.45 a.m. to go to the Churchill Transplant Centre. A Sunday had been selected so nobody could criticise us for wasting NHS resources. This was a very humbling day, thirty people, nurses, technicians, anaesthetists, operating department assistants and surgeons assembled for the pre theatre huddle, all giving freely of their time and effort. Prior to the huddle we met the donor and recipient, and their family. This, as might be expected, was quite emotional. A long day ensued with surgery by Isabel and me. We were lucky to have Cesar Diaz Garcia, one of the surgeons at the original Swedish series, with us, giving us great encouragement. Ben and Saal as always provided great support and insights. Our theatre Sister Jo was a tower of strength. Professors Friend and Sinha came in to wish us well. Retrieval of a good graft was achieved by the mid-afternoon, Isabel then left the explant to lead the back table work. Saal, Cesar and I finished the retrieval operation. We also had our collaborators, Liza Johannesson and Juliano Testa in Dallas available by phone, a facility much utilised and appreciated in that week. Venkatesha Udupa and Srdjan Saso meanwhile had commenced the preparation of the recipient. Once Isabel was happy with the back table work we moved to the implant procedure. There we removed two little vestigial uterine horns and Fallopian tubes leaving the vagina intact until later in the procedure. Isabel and Venkatesha then performed all the vessel join ups (anastomoses). We finished by opening the vagina and suturing the graft onto it. What a day, 21 hours in total. We had been phoning the family to keep them in the loop. We arrived back at the Cotswold Lodge at 6.30 a.m. on the Monday. I had adopted the Lille Bollinger approach that "I drink champagne when I'm happy and when I'm sad," and bought a bottle—sadly not Bollinger, a lot cheaper with me. We were exhausted but happy and must have been making some noise; the people above and next door thumped on my ceiling and wall! They probably thought we were drunk students. Students, yes; drunk, no.

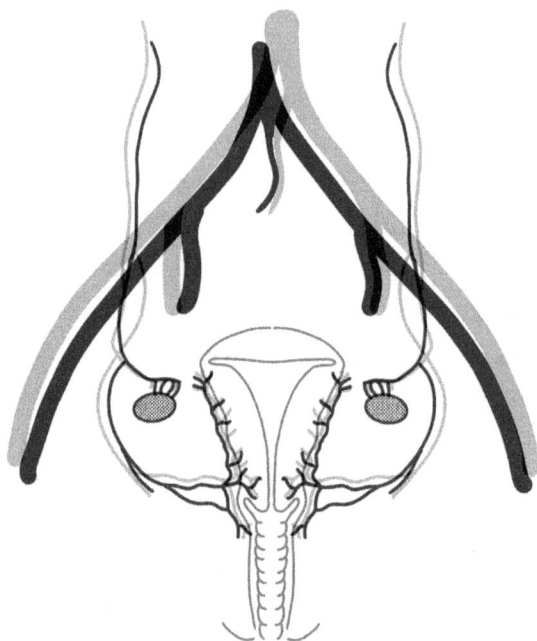

Fig 2: Implanted uterus graft

There followed an unbelievably stressful week where, again, the gynaecological and transplant skill mix gave us great strength but personal stress. Isabel, Saal and I were back in Gees restaurant on the Thursday night all agreeing we could do with counselling for PTSD. This was without doubt the most stressful week of my surgical career. We knew that from the point of implantation there is a 20% chance of the uterus having to be removed. We pored over the literature and by Wednesday, with normal scans of the uterus and vessels, the chance was probably down to 10%, by

Friday we had a cervical biopsy to check for rejection of the new organ, there was none, maybe down to 5% and one week later we had a second normal biopsy and our patient had a period. Wow, were we all happy; you remember earlier, if the transplanted uterus menstruates the chance of a successful pregnancy is very high. Four months later the donor and recipient have made an excellent recovery and the new womb is menstruating and normal on ultrasound scanning.

Never in the field of gynaecology was a period so much desired by so many for one woman. The two women and their families went through a huge event, always demonstrating good humour and great understanding. The extended Oxford team were stellar. The technician running the cell saver device to collect blood switched his machine on at 9.30 a.m. on the Sunday and switched it off at 5.30 a.m. the following morning. He, like the nursing and anaesthetic teams, were just amazing, the whole thing truly humbling. Since then Isabel, Ben and Saal have done much work to keep our patients safe in the post -operative phase, with much work ongoing to maintain optimal immunosuppression.

So Womb Transplant UK is finally a reality, 25 years after we first performed the procedure in the laboratory and, ironically, ten years to the exact day that the first Swedish procedure happened. Our team is well placed to have the world's biggest deceased donor programme due to the great organisational skills of NHS BT, and the next step is to produce a sustainable living donor programme too.

Looking to the future, I suspect around 2030, living and deceased donor and transplants will become quite routine. Endometrial transplants may happen from stem cell grown endometrium, or with PRP. There is still much work to be done before transplantation is likely to succeed in the transgender setting. By the 2040s we will have whole wombs grown from stem cells, and possibly after that, extracorporeal pregnancies.

I promised you earlier a plug for the charity and here it is: wombtransplantuk.org. Charity number 1138559 and go to "donate now." I can assure that our team intend to push at the boundaries of this area for many years to come. It's all part of "Never give up!"

Rule 2.

Never Say Never

If you don't try to help the patient you won't. What follows is a handful of stories relating to cancer care that have stuck with me through my many years as a surgeon. To me, they epitomise the resilience of the human spirit and show that, when the future seems bleak, just a glimmer of hope can be enough to see us through the darkest of times.

A middle-aged patient came to me via the pathologist Dr Ian Lindsay (pathologists perform analysis of tissue removed at surgery and also post-mortems). A GP some way out of London had a patient who had been "opened and closed" with a suspected ovarian cancer. The patient had gone to her doctor requesting a second opinion and she arrived at my consulting room. She was suffering much discomfort because of her watermelon-sized mass, with symptoms resulting from the pressure the mass was applying to her abdomen and its organs. She otherwise seemed fit and healthy and had brought scans with her. I agreed to review these at our weekly meeting with colleagues from all the branches of the cancer team—this is known as the multi-disciplinary meeting (MDT). We met the following week and I told her I thought it was removable with appropriate planning.

The patient and I duly agreed a date the following week for the surgery. On admission, she was seen by anaesthetist Dr Andrew Lawson (sadly deceased). Andrew picked up that there may have been a cardiac issue and cancelled the operation; a very smart move. Two weeks later the woman had re-plumbed coronary arteries with coronary stents and was duly booked on my list again. Two days before the operation I woke with a start at 4 a.m. In a moment of complete clarity, I realised that because of her cardiac risks she should be operated on in the Hammersmith hospital which, quite rarely for any hospital, performs both gynaecological cancer and cardiac surgery.

Of course, this was all happening in the run up to Christmas. I phoned the woman, apologised and the operation was rescheduled for the third of January. Safe to say, I had the most sober Scottish New Year I had had for many a year!

The third of January arrived and the patient was brought to the anaesthetic room, administered her anaesthetic and then, completely out of the blue, developed severe cardiac problems. Following prompt and lifesaving treatment by the anaesthetist, Dr Geoff Lockwood, rather than my gynaecological operating theatre, she was wheeled into the cardiac theatre where her coronary arteries were re-plumbed once again. It is important to note that there are very few hospitals where this immediate action could have been pulled off. Thank goodness for the Hammersmith. She survived and the operation was rescheduled.

To further complicate matters, she then developed renal failure requiring dialysis; this was because of the ever-growing mass compressing her kidneys and ureters. We yet again had to postpone her surgery. We were lucky Hammersmith hospital has renal dialysis facilities and she was admitted to the renal unit instead of the gynaecology ward preoperatively.

The common perception of surgeons is that we are an arrogant bunch, emotionally removed from our patient; this generally couldn't be further from the truth. We all worry a lot about our patients and I know, in this instance, I felt this woman deserved a break. We are all dealt a bad hand at some point in life, but this was right over the score. Unbelievably she managed to remain positive in the face of such adversity.

Finally, her surgery rolled round once again. I, as I always do, went to the ward to see her before theatre. This is always important— the patient's emotions are running high; anxiety, relief, excitement, fear, impatience. On that morning we exchanged a hug. We both knew that there was a 10 to 20% chance she wouldn't make it through the day. I don't normally hug my patients, but nor do I normally quote such dismal statistics.

Remarkably, despite the enormous size of the tumour, all the cancer, with the exception of one involved lymph node was confined within the ovary. She made it through.

The operation had involved removal of the uterus, Fallopian tubes, both ovaries, the omentum (fatty structure in the abdomen) and the pelvic and para aortic lymph nodes (alongside the aorta, the main vessel leading from the heart). Although the bowel was stuck to the outside, it was uninvolved and while the ureters (the tubes between the kidneys and the bladder) were compressed they were not involved in the cancer. She made an excellent post-operative recovery. Normally with an involved lymph node (lymph node metastasis), chemotherapy is used but this isn't and wasn't possible for somebody on dialysis, so for this woman the treatment stopped here. Even more remarkably, a few months later her kidneys started working again spontaneously and she no longer required dialysis. There was much speculation as to whether chemotherapy should be instituted so many months post-surgery when all the scans said she was in complete remission. I know the first year she took her whole family on a cruise, and recently we spoke so I could ask her permission to tell you this story—she said yes, and is still in fine fettle. She sends me a Christmas card every year. This isn't just a card from an old patient but a reminder that, above all else, hope prevails and she really epitomises the maxim 'never say never.'

I know that I have been extremely fortunate to have worked at Imperial College Healthcare NHS Foundation Trust, London, over the years at St Mary's, the Chelsea and Westminster, Charing Cross, Queen Charlotte's and the Hammersmith hospitals. It is amazing to work on the theatre corridor at the Hammersmith surrounded by expert gynaecological cancer surgeons, hepato-biliary and cardio-thoracic surgeons as well as transplant surgeons. This allows our hospital to perform very complex multi-team surgery, all in an atmosphere of harmony and collaboration with an amazing group of can-do nursing staff. Many of these colleagues have invented novel procedures, it is a truly brilliant place to work.

A classic example of this 'never say never' team working happened a few years ago now. A woman in her late twenties was referred to my colleague, medical oncologist Professor Michael Seckl, and myself, with a type of tumour called a teratoma. These arise in the ovaries and generally behave in a benign fashion. They are, in fact, the most common complex tumours to affect young women and are also called dermoid cysts or mature teratomas. They arise from eggs and normally, when mixed with sperm, become babies. These germ cell tumours therefore often contain teeth, hair, brain tissue, skin—all the constituents of a human being. I removed a huge 25 cm tumour many years ago which, when analysed by Dr Ian Lindsay, was found to have so much neural tissue that he declared it larger than a human brain. These tumours can be benign, which are known as mature teratomas, or cancerous, which are called immature teratomas.

The woman who presented that morning had a mature, benign teratoma but it was behaving very aggressively. It was in both her ovaries, in balls round her abdomen and pelvis; it also occupied a large proportion of her liver and was growing through her diaphragm and the lower lobe of her right lung.

She was the mother of four young children and also her husband's carer, since he was seriously physically debilitated. The woman was terrified, having been told she was inoperable.

When we looked at the scans the pelvic and abdominal disease looked removable, but we reckoned that the liver and the lung looked much harder. At this point entered a bigger team—Professor Long Jiao, hepato-biliary surgeon and Mr John Anderson, cardiothoracic surgeon. They reviewed the liver, lung and the lesions growing through the diaphragm and declared these sites of disease removable. One thing was certain, it was going to be a long day in the operating theatre.

The patient was understandably terrified of this surgery. The alternative, however, was death. The day of the operation came and I assisted Long, who opened the abdomen. He isolated the blood supply to the half of the liver with the tumour and John was then called. He incised the chest and split the sternum open. Dr Geoff Lockwood, the anaesthetist, (it's handy he is both a gynaecological and thoracic anaesthetist) collapsed the patient's right lung. John then detached the lower lobe of the lung with the tumour in it. He cut out half the diaphragm and part of the pericardium, the membrane round the heart. I have to confess to being slightly traumatised, having not seen the inside of a chest since houseman days. Long then returned and, with another clever device, cut the liver in two. Out came the tumour, with half the liver, one lobe of lung and the diaphragm in one single sample. It was unbelievable. I looked on, gobsmacked at what my fellow surgeons had pulled off. John put in a plastic diaphragm, wired the sternum and closed the chest. Long then closed the hepatic and abdominal incisions. She was my patient, but that day my role was very much that of assistant. We all took the decision that she had

had enough for one day and my part would wait for another two to four weeks to let her recover.

Two weeks later she was readmitted and it was time for me to attempt to rid her of the remining tumour. I opened her abdomen and removed her uterus, Fallopian tubes, ovaries and various balls of tumour including the final one which was attached to her spleen, necessitating removal of that organ—another colleague, Angus McIndoe helped with this. Yet again this was proving to be more complicated than I had bargained for.

Incredibly, the woman recovered astoundingly quickly. There were no post-operative complications and she was fighting fit in no time. More importantly, she remains well to this day many years later with no recurrence of her terrible tumour. The point of this story is the enormous value of extended team work and what a privilege it is to have such great colleagues; that theatre corridor at Hammersmith is just an amazing place to work in.

Both these stories epitomise the golden rule in cancer care, "Never say never," and both brave women and their surgical teams lived up to it.

Rule 3.

Be flexible — Adapt to situations as they develop and do not presume to sit in moral judgement

Back in the late eighties, I undertook a thesis on the interaction of HIV-related immunosuppression and cervical cancer. During this time, I was working at St Mary's Hospital in West London. For three years, I looked after a group of fifty women infected with HIV. My role wasn't just to investigate whether HIV caused cervical cancer, but was to look after them as whole people to the best of my ability. Here was a group of young women infected with this dreadful virus which, at the time, killed everybody that got it. I also had a control group of fifty HIV negative women who were matched for age, smoking and approximate number of lifetime sexual partners. To care for these women and to encourage their participation in the study I offered an on-call service during the day for the group, in case any of them developed emergencies.

I, in addition, had one male patient, a Scotsman. His girl-friend was also my patient and they both were infected with HIV. This was in the days before effective treatment for the virus. They were tragic times and virtually all of my patients died. By the mid-nineties, effective anti-retroviral treatment came along and everybody went back to a virtually normal life expectancy, not without inter current conditions. It was a bit like diabetes pre-insulin, everybody died until insulin came along (in the 1920s) and the prognosis changed forever, but not without its complications.

My solo male patient, who I will call Steve, used to turn up in my clinic asking for various medication and always for the sleeping tablet, temazepam. Temazepam, was widely available and you could aspirate the contents of the capsule with a needle and syringe, and then self-inject or share with a friend intravenously, known as jacking up, if you were so inclined. I forgot to say that 40% of my patients were intravenous drug users. Anyway, the rule always was NO temazepam and I would never prescribe it. I always got along well with this guy, partly because we were both from similar Scottish backgrounds. He undoubtedly was the black sheep of his family, the rest being respectable lawyers and teachers. I certainly knew a couple of folk from school who went badly off the rails with drugs. One of my bosses also commented that I got on well with the drug users because I had the same personality—I won't dispute I am of an addictive nature, but have kept it under reasonable control, and always stuck to legal substances.

Steve was known to carry a selection of weapons and had stuck a 6-inch blade through his case notes into the desk during a consultation with one of my bosses, who calmly replied, "You clearly are a little upset this morning."

On another morning, I was called by the Drug Dependency Unit (DDU) to say that his girlfriend was very sick and would I come and see her. The DDU was about 400 yards down the road from our clinic. I arrived at the building, which was like walking into a student party in Glasgow at 3 a.m. with lots of people lying around, their eyeballs rolled up. The difference here being it was 11 a.m. in an NHS facility. I was smartly dressed, with a jacket, collar and tie. As I walked in one woman looked up and said "Who are you, you poncy bastard?" Cue Steve, who had met me at the door.

"F**k off, you c**t, he's my doctor!"

That certainly had the desired effect. I then walked into the clinic room where his girlfriend was waiting. I asked a few questions, examined her and made the arrangements for immediate transfer to Almroth Wright ward, where she surely needed to be. I helped her out of the room to the staff who were going to take her to the ward. I then returned to the clinic room to finish my notes. In walked Steve—there were no seats for the patients in this room, only one for the doctor and a couch for the patient. Anyway, he lifted his shirt and produced a revolver.

"Is that f***ing thing loaded?" I asked.

"Yeah, there is no point in having a shooter without bullets, do you mind if I put it on the desk?" Steve replied.

I then said "I agree about the bullets and, er, yes please, putting it on the desk is a great idea."

Now I know this all sounds very laid back, but we have always been a shooting family and I am very familiar with guns. In addition, it never occurred to me that there was any personal threat to me. Steve then asked me for some temazepam.

"No way," I said, "you know the rules." Then I left, telling him I was off to the ward to check his girlfriend was okay.

What then happened I only knew of the following day when my clinic was interrupted by the head of security accompanied by a policeman.

"Richard,' said the policeman, 'did somebody produce a gun on you yesterday, in clinic at the DDU?"

"Yes," I replied.

'And did you call security?'

"No," I said, without hesitation.

'Are you used to people producing firearms in your clinic?"

"No,' I said again, 'but I knew there was no threat to me." I do remember the policeman shaking his head. They then explained what had happened after I left. Steve had called one of the outreach workers into the clinic room and asked him to prescribe temazepam, who said he wasn't a doctor and couldn't prescribe. At this point, Steve placed the gun in his ear, swung the revolving mechanism and asked him if it was his lucky day, à la Clint Eastwood in the Dirty Harry movies. This poor fellow still said he couldn't prescribe (at that point I think I would have done if I'd been him). Steve pulled the trigger and there was a dull click, no bullet, thanks be to God. As punishment, they closed the DDU, the poor outreach worker took time off and Steve was arrested. This story I hope demonstrates Adapting to a Changing Situation and treating the patient without moral judgement.

Continuing with this theme, I was at this time the gynaecologist to the West London Prostitutes Group—part of my research post. I may say I was the only male doctor ever invited to their Christmas party. They were a decent bunch of women, most of whom had been trapped into that life on arriving from the North of England and Scotland at Euston and King's Cross stations.

There was a classic morning where my connection with this group caused me some not inconsiderable embarrassment. I was doing my clinic accompanied by a young pre-clinical medical student. In those days, when studying medicine, for the first two to three years you were kept clear of patients and then in the last three years you were released on the unsuspecting public. During my first clinical attachment, a classmate was asked to listen to an attractive young woman's chest. He looked really nervous and then put his head between her breasts to get his ear on her chest. The consultant slapped the back of his head and suggested it was more customary to use a stethoscope!

My young student seemed pretty naïve, but Sexually Transmitted Infection (STI) clinics are not places you remain naïve for long. On that day I received a big brown package, which looked interesting amongst the boring mail. I eagerly ripped it open and out spilled a mound of pornographic magazines. Some of my patients had thought it would be very funny to send me this material as a joke. I was left red faced, stammering that I was the victim of a prank.

Returning to my HIV positive female patients the important thing to remember is that, in the face of so much suffering, some of these young women really wanted babies. I was twenty-eight years of age and finally began to understand the drive in many of my patients to start a family. At that time in the HIV world, medicine and morals were much mixed up. It was during this research period that the contentious issues around infertility first arose for me. At this time in the late 1980s, once a man or a woman was infected with HIV the average incubation from infection to development of full blown AIDS was ten to eleven years, and of course some progressed faster. Once AIDS developed, death was inevitable. During this time, these patients had to deal with all the uncertainties of their diagnosis, not knowing how long they would live or how they would die. However, they were like the cancer patient in remission, they were living with their disease; not dying of it yet, but with all the uncertainties in the face of a new disease.

These poor patients also had to suffer public opprobrium and fear, even from their nursing and medical carers. I well remember as a Registrar in Stobhill hospital, Glasgow, in 1986, performing a Caesarean section on an HIV-infected woman. When she walked to the labour ward there was a cleaner walking behind her, disinfecting the floor as she walked, quite unbelievable today. At that time, 25% of babies born to HIV-infected parents were infected themselves. We knew that much transmission happened at the time of delivery, hence Caesarean section was mandatory.

There was one shaft of humour on that day, however. There were no safety glasses to prevent splash injuries to the eyes so my assistant and I wore our Reactolite Rapide sunglasses—these, for the record, were aviator design. The patient and staff were all laughing as the cool surgical team set to work; it was important not to look up at the theatre lights! It all worked out well and mother and baby made a good recovery, the baby being uninfected with the virus.

In the late 1990s, highly active antiretroviral therapy (HAART) arrived and the whole picture transformed. What had been a death sentence became a lifelong condition, as long as you took the medication. Thus, with HAART, patients could be rendered with no active virus, making them non-infectious to others and the chance of a woman transmitting the virus to her baby fell to 2% so the use of Caesarean section as a strategy to prevent transmission to the baby became questionable.

When it came to HIV infection and infertility there were three groups. The first was HIV infected men with HIV negative partners. If they had sex to try for a baby they could infect their partner and, prior to highly active antiretroviral therapy, there were no options for these men until in the early 90s when Augusto Semprini invented the technique of sperm washing in Milan. This was a standard IVF laboratory technique whereby the sperms swam out of the seminal fluid. The HIV virions (infectious particles) were in the fluid, not attached to the sperms.

This was a stroke of pure genius on Augusto's part. I went to visit him in Milan, and a memorable visit it was. I was at a conference and phoned him asking to meet. He said he would send his two most beautiful medical students to collect me, which he duly did. They whisked me away to Augusto's hospital. He was in his office, in an immaculate white coat, shaped Armani-style. His office was very stylish and when he offered me a drink, his secretary opened a large cupboard which proved to be a drinks fridge full of Peroni beer, Prosecco and soft drinks. This made my office and entertainment facilities back in London look rather shabby, to say the least. On a very happy note this meeting led later to Augusto coming to the Chelsea and Westminster hospital in London and setting up the UK's first and only sperm washing service. This was done in conjunction with Carole Gilling Smith, IVF consultant and Simon Barton, Chief of the HIV service, Europe's largest; the process took five years from the Milan meeting until the first couples were treated.

The other two groups of HIV fertility patients were first where both the man and the woman were infected, so the only factor to consider was the 25% risk to the baby. This may seem small, but when faced with the odds the risk feels huge and so couples were deterred from having babies.

The final group was where the woman was infected but the man was not. Thus, there was a risk of transmission from woman to man during unprotected sex as well as risk to the baby, once again of 25%. It is important to point out that an infected man could not transmit to a baby without first infecting the mother.

This was where much dispute broke out; I believed that it was very much the couple's right to evaluate the risk and decide, but for the HIV-negative man and his infected female partner, possibly we could render some assistance. This was in the form of sterile pots and syringes to allow the man to ejaculate into the pot, the semen could then be sucked up with a syringe and the contents inserted into the upper vagina—hey presto, risks of infection to the man, sorted!

I was proposing to give out "the gear" to allow this when trouble broke out. Respected colleagues were unhappy about this proposed intervention; the argument was that we were potentially increasing the number of babies in the world infected with HIV. I took myself off to a Pharmacy in St John's Wood, a very upmarket area in North West London. I was wearing a tee shirt, shorts and boots. Remember, I am from Glasgow with the accent that accompanies that great city. For the St John's Wood pharmacist, at first sight, with my request for sterile syringes, pots and quills, I looked like the local drug dealer. That was exactly the initial supposition but when I told him I intended to fertilise my girlfriend without having sex with her, he smiled, admitting that in his experience this was a unique request. He did, however, agree to sell me "the gear." I then told him the story. What this proved was that any couple could follow this path without having been advised to and thereby protect the man from infection. For me, then, this followed corollary, so was it any way ethical to withhold this advice? Answer: No, I think not.

A few years ago, I was practising as a consultant at the Chelsea and Westminster hospital, in West London. I was looking after many women who came from the Royal Brompton National Heart hospital with their congenital heart disease. Many of them had been advised by the redoubtable Dr Jane Somerville that if they became pregnant and wished to go on to have a baby they would have a 50% chance of death. This proved little deterrent to many, and the mortality rate was, indeed, 50%. Contrast this with a study published at much the same time, (mid-90s) which surveyed women having nuchal fold scans to determine the risk of their baby having Down's syndrome. This is where the skin on the back of the baby's head is measured and it gives a reliable risk of Down's syndrome so as to determine if more invasive tests on the baby are required. These invasive tests are inevitably riskier to the mother and baby. The idea behind the nuchal fold programme was to determine babies at a greater risk than 1 in 200 (nowadays 1 in 150) thus allowing those women to go on and have invasive tests (e.g. Chorion villous sampling, cordocentesis or amniocentesis). However, the survey showed that women in East London regarded a risk of greater than 1 in 800 to their baby as unacceptable; this made a mockery of the scheme in many ways. However, the vital fact here is, for a woman that wishes to have children, her perception of risk for herself in having a baby versus the acceptable risk to her baby: 50% mortality in the mother is OK, but almost 0.01% is the acceptable figure of risk for the baby. I don't know that there is any data with respect to men and these sort of statistics, I suspect not, but as a man I believe you would find few men prepared to risk a

50% mortality in pursuit of a baby—they might well be prepared to accept that risk in protection of their young once born, but I doubt on the basis of a baby as a future concept.

With much of my work over the years, people from all walks of life have stated that women who are prepared to risk their lives with fertility-sparing surgery for cancer, sub optimal treatment for HIV back in the 90s, or those seeking uterine transplantation must be ignorant or foolish. In my experience, they are neither. Almost all of the women I have seen and cared for are fit to plead and just have that natural desire for many, namely to have children.

I want to tell you a final story in a slightly different vein, but that does fit neatly into our chapter title—don't sit in moral judgement, be flexible in your approach. I was a junior doctor in Glasgow Royal Infirmary back in the mid-eighties and on call late at night. We were always being called to wards with elderly patients with uterine prolapse—this is where the uterus falls completely out of the vagina. It is remedial by surgery or, in the very elderly, a ring pessary. These are essentially tough rubber rings in various sizes that sit in the vagina and hold everything up. So common were these calls from around the hospital that I, and my fellow gynaecologists, carried a selection in my white coat pocket—yes we did wear them back then, often with a carnation in the button hole.

One evening, I appeared late on a psychogeriatric ward. There was a very helpful nurse who agreed to accompany me to the patient. No history was possible, no dialogue was possible but, on examination, the patient's uterus was lying in the bed. The standard technique is to reinsert the uterus through the vagina, open one's index and middle fingers which allows you to assess the size of the ring required. The patient wasn't particularly cooperative, but with the assistance of the staff nurse we managed to replace the uterus. However, as I was assessing the size, the patient came out with the immortal line, "Get out of there, there's been nobody in there since the war." That was the end of that—consent was officially withheld, and the nurse and I retired, laughing a lot, I have to confess.

I do hope these stories illustrate flexibility in the face of changing situations and just how important having a baby is for some women. HIV is happily a transformed disease, although not without ongoing issues; it is easy to forget how terrible it was pre HAART. Come what may our job is to help, be that infertility, or ring pessaries and not judge but respond to the patient's needs and wishes.

Rule 4.

Always tell the truth and never tell lies. "How long have I got doctor?" — take great care with prognostication

This story relates to what happens with poor prognostication and the pitfalls of trying to guess how long somebody will live. I was sitting in my clinic at Chelsea and Westminster many years ago when a couple I knew came in to see me. Let me paint you a picture. The woman, usually warm and engaging, stared at the floor and made no eye contact. Her husband, who was typically a charming man, looked upset and slightly aggressive. This sense was accentuated by the fact that he had to stand because of a bad back. The act of standing when others are sitting doesn't make for everybody's psychological comfort. I felt some unease in the pit of my stomach.

"How are you?" I asked.

She responded with a blank stare at the floor. I asked again, still no reply. I tried a different tack.

"Has something or somebody upset you?"

Silence. I looked to the husband to gauge his response, he raised his eyebrows. This consultation was going from bad to worse.

"Did something happen at the last consultation to cause you upset?" Again, no response. Then the husband gave a slow nod.

"I have moved over to the other side," the woman said.

I looked at her and thinking I understood her meaning, replied "If I understand you correctly, I don't think you are on the other side, or close to it."

Now it's important to mention that this woman had been a patient of mine for some years and her cancer had been managed by surgery at least twice. She had also had chemotherapy on two occasions. However, at this time we thought she was again in remission. She was almost certainly going to recur, but we were in no position to determine when that might be. I asked what had been said at the last consultation. The husband replied that she had been told she had two months to live and it was now three months later and she was still alive. I asked who had told her this, to which she replied with the name of an excellent young junior doctor; highly skilled and destined to have a bright future, but inexperienced in his consultations. It all started to make sense. I imagined the scenario went something like this:

Patient: "How long have I got?"

Doctor: "I don't know"

The patient and her family inevitably push harder for an answer. The young doctor prevaricates a little further and is pushed once again.

Patient: "Can you give me just a rough time frame?"

Doctor: "I really couldn't say..."

Upon being pushed once more for an answer under ever increasing pressure, he drags a figure from thin air, in this case; two months. Little could he have realised the catastrophe of such a guess. The patient returned home and immediately summoned her family from round the world to visit before she died. Even more tragically she had asked them to come when her death had been predicted. Of course, she was perfectly alive and the family then returned to their homes. From then on, she had "died" in her own mind and resigned herself to the fact that it was only a matter of time before her passing.

It's important at this point to say that this woman looked perfectly healthy. In my view, she was likely to live for many months, if not years. Of course, I could be wrong and what if I said I thought she would last for months and then she died suddenly? She did, however, look well enough for me to tell her with confidence that I thought that she did not look like she was dying and with that she finally made eye contact. However, it was obvious she did not believe me. I asked to examine her and asked a few clinical questions, to which she agreed. I asked her to look at he mirror beside me, and asked her if she looked any more like she was dying than I did? I did now manage to lighten things a little by telling her I reckoned I was very healthy, or at least hoped so. This brought at least the hint of a smile. I then excused myself to get the specialist nurse to come and help. We agreed a plan with the patient and her husband that admitted that we were unsure of her prognosis but did not think that anything untoward was happening at this time. However, we also admitted that we might be wrong and that what was required were further investigations to confirm that things were OK. She was so distressed that we arranged for her admission to Annie Zunz ward, the gynaecology ward at Chelsea and Westminster hospital. She spent two days in hospital and, happily, her CT scans and blood tests were all normal. On the ward, the nursing and medical staff did their usual fantastic job of putting a smile on people's faces. She went home a changed woman.

The cure? No surgery, no treatment, just good old-fashioned communication; the progenitor of the problem of course being old-fashioned bad communication.

So, is there a better way to explain the uncertainties? Can we be honest when asked that question "How long have I got, doctor?" I think we can.

The 4-cusp approach to cancer care

With my colleagues, medical oncologist Dr Mark Bower and specialist nurse Catherine Gillespie, I developed this approach to patient care over many years of sitting in clinics explaining to patients where they are with their cancer, not just in physical terms but conceptually in relation to their cancer and their life expectancy and its quality. The four cusps (A, B, C, D) which I am about to briefly explain, bear no relationship to the stages of cancer (I, II,

III, & IV). Stages of cancer refers to how far a cancer has spread and in gynaecology the classification always involves four stages, I being the earliest where the cancer is confined to the organ that the cancer is arising from, Stages II and III means there has been further spread and stage IV distant metastasis. Below is the pictorial model which I draw to assist with explaining to patients their prognosis. The four cusps are A "cured," B "living with cancer," C pre-terminal, D dying. The reason for the inverted commas is that we have no certainty as to what will happen to any patient until five years has elapsed; this is the huge conundrum for the person with cancer. For all patients, the goal is to achieve what is called complete remission. This means there is no detectable disease left in the patient by any of our tests. The big question is, is it going to come back?" If it is, "When is that going to happen? Or is it never going to happen? In which case the patient is truly cured. For gynaecological cancers, at the end of five years if there has been no recurrence, you can count yourself cured – no inverted commas here. This is referred to as the cured circle. This nomenclature has been shown to be psychologically important for patients and families.

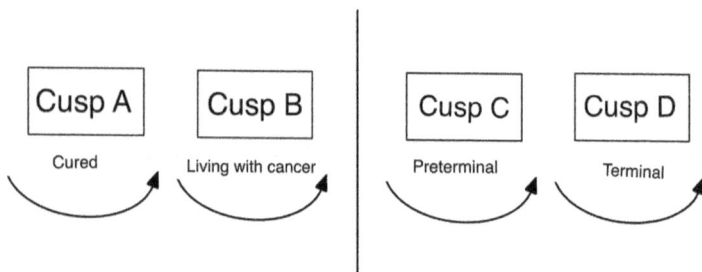

Fig 3. 4 Cusps

This pictorial representation or 'map' to having cancer has seemed to resonate with patients and their families. I think that, perhaps, symbols can represent concepts that are difficult with language. In the words of St Thomas Aquinas, "man cannot understand without images."

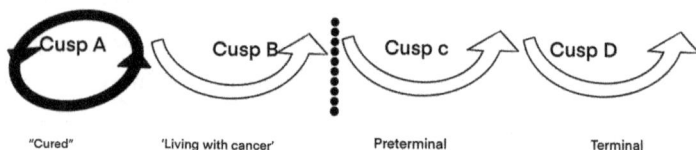

Fig 4. Cusp A: Five years after diagnosis, the patient enters the "cured" circle.

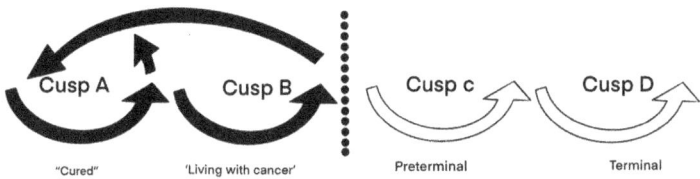

Fig 5 Cusp B: The patient living with cancer following surgery, chemo-therapy and radiotherapy, enters the "cured" circle after 5 years.

The two most important aspects of the 4-cusp pictorial model are. the action of folding it down the central line and the "circle" aimed at in both cusps A and B.

Folding the paper and thus dispatching Cusp C and D to being "out of sight," coupled with the powerful image of a circle suggesting "holism" are the model's strongest features. Most patients, on being told their cancer diagnosis, jump to the conclusion that they have been given a death sentence. Much of the remainder of the consultation will be forgotten, the patient only remembering the diagnosis itself. The first thing I am able to tell the vast majority of my patients is that they are not pre-terminal or dying, in other words in Cusps C and D but either in cusp A— cured—where we think the chances of recurrence are less than 10% or B—living with cancer—where the patient has had surgery and chemotherapy or radiotherapy or all three. This was the situation the last women was in. She had recurred twice but was disease free at the time she asked "how long have I got?"

The pictorial image for her was this:

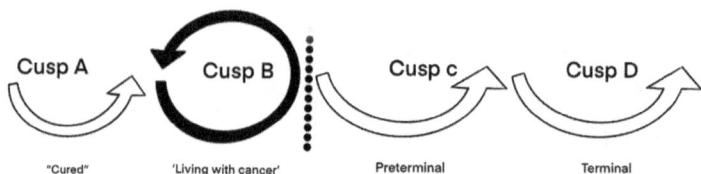

Fig 6: Four Cusps: "living with cancer, stuck in the "living with cancer circle" and very unlikely to ever be cured.

So, for this patient, the better approach would have been to produce a drawing like the one above, tell her cure was almost impossible but that we had no idea when she would tip into being preterminal. Folding the paper down the middle dotted line seems to be helpful psychologically and puts Cusps C and D literally out of sight and, to a degree, out of mind.

All of us are different and every cancer is different, but it is important in the first instance to be aware that over 50% of gynaecological tumours are cured in the long term. The death sentence outlook is just not true for most people.

No doctor is likely, if he/she has any sense, to answer the question 'How long have I got?' directly, since they do not and cannot know the answer. This is why they are much more likely to answer using a variant of the 4-cusp approach to cancer care—this is not obfuscation but truth. This approach is patient-centred and allows the patient to see where they are with their disease. I have spent many years drawing pictures for patients showing them which operation they are going to have. Rarely has the picture been taken away for future reference. This may be because of the quality of my artwork, or it may be that people get the message. On the other hand, the "4 cusp" diagram has been taken away by numerous patients to assist in further dialogue with their families. To me the most amazing thing is how often this scrap of paper has been produced years later from people's wallets; it is always still folded.

But of course, there are tragic story when events run the other way. This doesn't happen very often, but we cannot deny that sometimes it does. I need to tell this story to maintain the balance and to bring home the pitfalls of prognostication. Patients have on occasion, come in to clinic, unfolded the paper, and said "I think sadly I have arrived" in cusp C. Even here, the model has proven useful, since to me, this is always the hardest conversation one ever has.

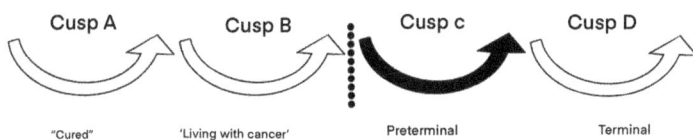

Fig 7. Cusp C-Pre terminal where treatment is symptom orientated and not aimed at cure or prolongation of life.

I had a patient who had gone through her treatments for ovarian cancer, she was out the other side of her surgery and chemotherapy by a good few months and all was going well; she was in complete remission. We sat together on a Friday morning in the Charing Cross clinic; we talked the cusps, she was firmly in Cusp B, cure was possible, although recurrence and re-treatment at some point more likely. I arranged to see her in three months.

To my horror, I was phoned on the Monday, three days later, to be told she had died suddenly from a rare metastasis, in fact this is only the second time in my career I have ever encountered it. This was a rare event but truly awful. Contrary to popular belief, things usually in our field do not go wrong quickly, but on this occasion, they did, and it was a terrible shock for all of us.

Finally I do wish to recount to you a story from my days in obstetrics, many years ago now, but this so demonstrates the need to be truthful, even in the face of political correctness. A woman in her thirties was pregnant with her first baby. I had seen her in the antenatal clinic on and off through her pregnancy along with the midwives; she was planning a home water birth. It was noted when she was at 34 weeks gestation that her baby was breach.

Now, quite rightly, over the next few weeks she was checked to see if the baby had turned to head first. By 39 weeks it had not. Week on week I had said all the right things, explained the risks to her and her baby of her proposed mode of delivery. This, rightly, was always couched in non-judgemental terms. However, at the 39 week visit, I further emphasised the risks she was running to no effect upon the plan. At the end of that Friday morning antenatal clinic, I returned upstairs to my office where I contemplated my counselling for her over a sandwich. I was suddenly struck by the fact that, while if anything went wrong my notes and advice were unimpeachable, I had never actually said what I really thought and came to the conclusion that was morally wrong in this circumstance. I knew if I did tell her what I really thought I could be in terrible trouble, but to fail in this duty of being candid would be the bigger failure. So guess what? I picked up the phone, dialled her number and she picked up.

"I'm sorry to phone you"

"Is everything OK doctor?"

"Yes and no" says I. "Everything I have said to you has been true and correct but I haven't told you what I actually think."

"Oh how do you mean?"

"Honestly, I think your birth plan is crazily dangerous for you and your baby"

"What would you do, doctor?"

I replied, "An elective Caesarean section as soon as possible."

She was sitting with her husband, they conferred and she then replied "I'll have the Caesarean, when?" I asked her when she had last eaten, and she told me she had just had breakfast.

"Let's deliver your baby this afternoon."

This we duly did with a healthy mother and baby as the outcome. The woman and her family, mercifully, were not only happy with the outcome but thanked me for my honesty. I bring this story in to demonstrate how easy it is to be led astray by one's environment into doing the wrong thing, and the importance of sticking to the truth as you see it.

This chapter starts by illustrating the dangers of prognostication, and then demonstrates the 4-cusp approach, which is a truthful model taking into account all the uncertainties of trying to predict the pathway of an individual woman's disease. The last account again illustrating the absolute requirement for truth even when it doesn't suit the dialogue of the time.

Rule 5.

Hit them hard and hit them fast – your first go at treating the patient is your best go

This is a slightly enigmatic golden rule, let me explain. If you ask anybody "If you were diagnosed with cancer how quickly would you want it dealt with?" The answer universally would be "Yesterday!" This is an understandable emotion, but not necessarily a right thinking approach. There are a few tumours which genuinely do grow really quickly and need to be managed as a matter of great haste, however most grow more slowly and a gap of a few weeks from symptoms to diagnosis to treatment is probably the right timing. Certain levels of wait are likely to be harmful, hence the NHS guidelines surrounding the two week wait process. This has been one of the little jewels in the crown of the NHS, introduced about twenty years ago. The idea was remarkably simple and all the better for it. If a patient went to their doctor with a wide range of symptoms e.g. bleeding from the vagina after the menopause, then a letter was to be faxed to the "2 week wait fax machine," which has more recently become an email. Thus, for the cost of a designated fax machine a new system appeared and it worked.

The whole concept of general practice being the gatekeeper to hospital based care is mostly successful. It works so well for conditions like asthma, diabetes, high blood pressure and cancers with obvious and predictable symptoms. It is however very difficult for the GP to gauge the vague symptoms associated with ovary cancer; tummy pains, abdominal distension, bloating, discomfort, these are things we all get. Sadly, but understandably, there are few women diagnosed with advanced ovarian cancer who do not feel at least somewhat aggrieved with their time from first complaining of symptoms until their diagnosis. Often there are no symptoms until the disease has spread and, even then, many of the symptoms are very mild and vague. This is why ovarian cancer has the reputation of being a silent killer.

A far more complicated system has since emerged, with various times that one can wait for diagnosis and treatment stipulated. This, as you might imagine, has created a large supporting bureaucracy, but on the whole it works well. Patients are taken through a system whereby they are referred in a timely fashion, they have their investigations, scans, biopsies etc. and then they have their surgery or chemotherapy or radiotherapy in good time thus minimising their chances of further disease spreading.

Virtually every time I sit with a patient at the start of their cancer journey I say to them, "We have a golden rule with cancer, hit it hard and hit it fast!" I will confess I copied this golden rule from the redoubtable Dr Mark Glazer, Consultant in Clinical Oncology. I guess it appeals also to the Glaswegian side of my personality. I vividly remember as a houseman in Glasgow in the eighties there was a lot of violence in hospitals. Patients were regularly assaulting or attempting to assault nursing and medical staff.

In response, a fair few patients were assaulted themselves, under the circumstances often pertaining this was probably right and proper. I do remember a management memo telling us that if we thought we were going to be hit, it was ok to hit first—a very Glasgow approach. When I was a student in Accident and Emergency, always the most dangerous place in the hospital, a patient hit one of the nurses in front of the waiting room. A group of men who were waiting to be seen dragged the fellow outside declaring they would make him a real casualty; they did.

So, what do we mean by this rule and why do we have to modify it?

Fundamentally, in a simple world it would be right, but this world isn't straightforward. If you are faced with a woman whose cancer is doubling every 24 hours and you are forced to remove that woman's uterus as soon as possible, she will be psychologically scarred. Everything seems to be going OK at the time of the emergency and the surgery. The patient goes home and returns at the two week visit to get the results, all is usually going well, then the six week visit arrives. The poor woman cannot get her head round the disaster of fertility loss and the speed with which it all happened. In my early days in private practice I would often meet patients who wanted things to happen at breakneck speed, one learns quickly that you only acquiesce to this sort of request for strictly medical reasons. A two to three week gap, from meeting to surgery with at least two meetings in this process, is far more likely to deliver the right results both physically and psychologically in the long term.

In addition, if you are looking after somebody who wishes to retain their fertility or some aspects of it, then further discussion of options and perhaps aspects of fertility care need to happen. An example would be retrieval of eggs for freezing prior to any treatment. This leads into the rule "Hit it hard."

Almost without exception, as soon as you do anything to preserve fertility you compromise on this rule. If we take the example of ovarian cancer we sometimes are able, in early disease, to remove only one ovary along with taking biopsies, leaving the other ovary and the uterus behind. The traditional approach was always to remove everything. We now know that the chances of the uterus giving trouble at a later date is very low, but the chance of cancer in the other ovary not visible on scanning sits at a variable percentage, depending on tumour type. It is usually a low chance, but devastating when it happens; this leads to complex consultations. If you have both ovaries removed and keep your uterus you can have babies using donated eggs from either a relative or an anonymous donor, a further layer of complexity, all compromising our golden rule.

So, while we started with "Hit them hard and hit them fast" but this might be better phrased "Hit them hard and fast some of the time but, maybe not quite so hard and fast most of the time."

Rule 6.

Never say "There is nothing more we can do". There always is, ask the patient how they feel. Do not presume to know the patient's desires

I vividly remember, as a medical student, being taught by the renowned Professor Sir Kenneth Calman. He told the wonderful anecdote of looking after a woman who was dying of her cancer. Calman taught me many things, but this lesson I have carried with me through my entire professional career. He taught us that the vital question to ask the patient is "Is there anything we can do for you that would help?" His patient replied "I would love to have my hair done, the full works. Cut, blow dry, style. I want to feel like me, for just a moment." Of course, Calman arranged it and, so the rumour went, also paid for it. This kind act made a huge difference to the patient's well-being. It's the little things that count. This lesson is so important and I will illustrate it with two examples of my own.

I used to do my main ward round of the week at the Chelsea and Westminster hospital on a Tuesday late afternoon. I duly arrived in the ward to be taken in to a side room where a new patient I had never met before had been admitted. The sense of anger in the room was palpable. The poor woman had a recurrence of her cervical cancer. It had previously been treated with chemotherapy and radiotherapy and had now returned creating a hole (fistula) between the bladder and the vagina. She also had involved para aortic lymph nodes. This combination made surgery, chemotherapy and radiotherapy all impossible. To put it as simply as possible – her options were extremely limited and, tragically, her life would soon come to an end. I presumed to think her anger related to this. As I approached her, I said "I know you are very angry and I think I know why, but can you tell me why?"

"I have been told there is nothing more can be done for me," she said, with a fiery look on her face.

I replied, "I haven't ever said that to you, I'm sorry to ask you again but what is making you feel so angry?"

She looked at me, I could see the anger rising, then she shouted "It's obvious, bloody obvious! I know it, you know it! We all know it!"

I hesitated before asking but knew I had to, so I did.

"What is obvious?"

Then came the totally unexpected reply.

"I smell of piss."

Oh, my goodness. That was not where I thought this was going. I was then able to reply "I can't personally do anything but I know a clever radiologist downstairs who I reckon can help."

The following day she went down to the X-ray department and an interventional radiologist inserted a tube directly through her back into the kidneys, thus allowing the urine to drain into bags strapped to her legs. Result! The patient went home and spent the next few weeks socialising with friends, eating out and enjoying normal life. A few weeks later she was readmitted. The seething anger was gone and I was met with peaceful, contented woman. Twenty-four hours later, she passed away.

Another example relates to a woman who was dying in our ward at the Chelsea and Westminster hospital. We had an unusual arrangement there. Most gynaecological wards are essentially surgical wards. At Chelsea and Westminster, Annie Zunz ward had patients having minor diagnostic procedures, major surgery, chemotherapy and palliative care. This was as a result of Sister Giselle Li In Oy's drive to total patient care. The result was that many patients chose to die in our ward rather than at home or in the hospice. They felt safe and cared for there, which they most assuredly were. I used to often sit with the palliative care patients, many of whom I had known for years. In palliative care, our question is somewhat simpler. "In the knowledge that we can't stop your disease, is there anything we could do for you that we are not already doing?" I posed this question to a very upset, dying patient. She looked at me with great anguish and I was apprehensive of her reply.

"I don't think there is anything you can do. I'm stuck in here dying and I don't know what to do."

"Try me," I responded.

"In my house, in my loft there are papers. Papers which need to be burnt! They need to be destroyed before I can go."

This was certainly a call to action. It wasn't our business to pry and platitudes were not going to work.

"Let me go and talk to Sister and see if anything can be done."

I duly talked to Giselle and she arranged for a staff nurse to accompany the patient home in an ambulance, the papers were retrieved from the loft and duly burnt. The patient returned to Annie Zunz ward and died within a day or two; she had been hanging on in psychological torment and had been unable to let go. At peace at last, she was able to pass.

These accounts of course focus on end of life care and I think show that doctors, nurses, relatives and friends have much to contribute and much suffering can be alleviated by listening to what the patient desires, rather than projecting their own.

Rule 7.

If you are the patient, don't lie to your nearest and dearest; if you are the nearest and dearest, don't lie to the patient

When you look at this Golden Rule in the cold light of day, it sounds obvious. You would be amazed how often it isn't so obvious to patients and their relatives in the thick of the cancer battle. We all have a natural desire to protect our nearest and dearest from hurt and harm. As doctors, we don't want to upset our patients but as professionals we have a duty to be truthful.

In the family, there is no professional relationship, usually caring and love, but of course, that's not universal. The strains of the cancer journey sadly split up many a family.

Personally, over the years, I have become more and more convinced that telling the truth is the only way. If lies are told, even for the best of motivations, they inevitably lead to more lies and later the discovery of those lies which leads to loss of trust. To illustrate this from a number of different angles, I want to recount to you some examples of where it has gone wrong.

A charming woman in her fifties came to see me with an ovarian cancer, which appeared to be quite advanced. We discussed the standard management which was to perform surgery and remove as much of the disease as possible, and to follow this with chemotherapy. After a number of visits to clinic I was unable to convince this woman to have surgery, chemotherapy or even discuss her condition with her family. In her case she had no husband, partner or children. She had an elderly mother. She was in a very bad place and rightly thought that her mother would be very upset. This type of situation doesn't arise very often and is always very frustrating to watch. We usually bring the patient back to clinic every few weeks with more tests in the hope the patient will come round before it's too late. In this woman's case, about four months after I first met her she decided to go for the surgery. She was a bit sicker than when she had first presented but seemed fit enough to withstand the surgery. We duly went to theatre and I opened her abdomen through a big incision from her bellybutton to her pubic area. To my horror on opening her up, her insides, bowels and pelvic organs were almost black in colour. The poor woman had left it too late, to touch anything now would lead to disaster. I had never seen anything quite like it. There followed a discussion with the surgical, anaesthetic and nursing team in that theatre and we all agreed that to continue was futile. The patient's abdomen was therefore closed and she was taken to recovery. She woke up completely but was clearly in a very bad way. I talked her through what we had found. She asked for a priest to be sent for, which was duly done. She asked me to phone her mother to tell her. The mother was at home, it was evening time and she lived outside the UK, so there was no chance of her getting there before the end. That was one of the worst calls I have ever had to make; a total bolt from the blue for the elderly mother, none of the things that should be said could have been said. The priest came and did the last rites in the recovery area of the operating theatre complex and the patient passed away. A total tragedy and much worse than it needed to be.

The opposite scenario of not talking to the patient but only to the relatives is, thankfully, a problem that has almost disappeared. I think this has come about because we all know that when we go to the doctor they are only meant to speak to the patient and must not speak to anybody else without the patient's specific permission.

I remember an elderly woman, aged ninety-eight. She was very charming, and totally sharp, in fact positively imperious. She came into hospital with vaginal bleeding. I took her to theatre and performed a hysteroscopy, looking inside her uterus, and discovered she had an early endometrial cancer. When I visited her on the ward after her minor procedure she was already dressed and sitting next to her bed ready to go home. All the other, much younger patients were still languishing in their beds. I sat down and told her that I felt pretty certain she had an early cancer. I said perhaps we should think about hormonal treatment to try to slow it up. She fixed me with a stare.

"What would you do if I was seventy-eight not ninety-eight?"

"Mm, I would offer you a hysterectomy. But there are risks with surgery which rise with age."

'I think I want the operation if you don't mind, doctor."

"Ok," says I, "Maybe we should have a chat with your daughter?"

"Doctor, may I remind you who is the patient, this is nothing to do with my daughter; I will be telling her my diagnosis, but you and I are making the decisions."

I had been well and truly put in my place. I looked at her sitting there ready to go home, she was a tough and highly likeable lady.

I smiled. "OK, it's a deal, we will confirm the analysis of what we have removed and schedule you for a hysterectomy in two weeks."

She thanked me and sure enough came in two weeks later for her operation. At that time patients stayed in hospital for five days after a hysterectomy. On her second post-operative day, I visited her on the ward to find her sitting next to the bed, fully dressed ready to go home. I saw her one more time in clinic, she was well. I explained our standard follow up of visiting for a check-up, every three months in the first year and every four months in the second, moving to six monthly check-ups for the next three years. She looked at me and said "I'm ninety-eight and you don't need me filling out your busy clinic. If I bleed again I'll come and see you." That was that, she went off with a smile and, I hope, lived for many more years, she sure had the right attitude.

Surgery in the elderly is interesting, the patient I described above still holds the record in my practice for oldest hysterectomy.

Over the years, attitudes have changed and below eighty years of age is no longer regarded as elderly. Many patients in their eighties undergo major surgery and the vast majority do very well. Once into the nineties, more caution is required. The rule of thumb is if you make it to that age, by definition you must be pretty tough. The surgery either tends to go very well, as described in the story above, or very badly—there is not much of a half-way house. It's funny and what I'm about to say may not seem very scientific, but if your patient is seventy and looks like they are eighty-five years old, they will behave as if they are eighty-five, and the opposite is also true. I guess it's down to the quality of collagen which determines how old we look and how we cope with the knife.

With the provision of translators in hospitals these days, the chance of the family hijacking a consultation is much less. It is why it's so important not to use family members and friends as translators except in extreme circumstances. I learned that particular lesson on Annie Zunz ward years ago.

There was an extremely sick patient admitted with advanced ovarian cancer. She, very unusually, was almost certainly beyond any treatment. I say very unusually because most cancer patients at diagnosis look normal. It's only in the terminal phase of cancer that people develop that terrible look which is the public image of cancer. I am aware that the image of the terminal cancer patient is in all of our mind's eyes because we have a relative or friend who we have known and have seen in their last days of their illness. Very, very few people first appear at their doctor looking like that. I went to talk to her only to discover she spoke no English

79

or French for that matter, the only two languages I can speak and my French is not brilliant (that's an understatement). She spoke some obscure language, which no staff on the ward spoke; but working in London we are not short of multi-linguists. At Hammersmith Intensive Care Unit, they have a map on the wall of the world with arrows to where the staff come from, answer: everywhere, how good is that? Brilliant, to my mind. No translator was immediately available. The situation required rectifying rapidly after what happened next. I started to explain the diagnosis in my usual direct fashion, with her family members offering translations as I spoke. The patient responded completely aberrantly, smiling and looking enthusiastic, she was either in denial or there was a totally false translation going on. Of course, it was the latter, and the family tried very hard to stop her knowing the truth. As you might expect she knew the score already in herself. When we all sat together with a translator, she and the family got to a place of truth, they were able to say the things that needed to be said and she passed peacefully a few days later.

The accounts in this chapter focus again on end of life care but again come back to the overarching theme that the truth will always out and better to start with it. Although at the beginning of the cancer journey the truth can be very difficult for the patient and her relatives, much heart ache can be prevented by utilising it. If all parties, the patient, her relatives, the doctors and the nurses all are truthful with each other trust is maintained, however difficult the circumstances.

Rule 8.

Understand personal humility: Doctors might be better doctors if they were patients themselves

The whole deal for professionals in any field is that we are meant to get it right all of the time. However, much as we all love to deny it, that just isn't always possible. My own experience is that whenever you think you've done something really smart, metaphorically speaking, God comes along and flicks your left testicle. The biggest juxtaposition of roles of course is when, as a doctor, you fall ill and have the unfortunate experience of becoming "the patient" - a very illuminating event indeed. The following accounts I regularly use with my patients. I usually start by saying "We are here to talk about you, not me, but I would like to tell you something that happened to me, which I think might help you."

Being a patient in a hospital is rarely a fun event. I often laugh with my patients that hospitals are full of people who would rather be somewhere else. Having said this, modern medicine has, to a degree, become dehumanising. It is vitally important that doctors keep to the old fashioned approach of taking a history—talk to the patient, understand their illness, but also their needs, desires and expectations. We then examine the patient and order the appropriate tests. There is a huge tendency these days to cut the corner to the tests, bypassing the history and examination. There is no doubting that the introduction of accurate ultrasound and a myriad of blood tests and other imaging techniques has vastly improved our abilities to treat patients effectively. It has short-ened hospital stays, many procedures that twenty years ago would keep a patient in hospital for a week or two now involve a day case procedure or one to two nights in hospital. These are all great advances but it has created a tendency for the patient to become a number, not a person. The desire for quick turnaround in all settings does have a dehumanising effect. Staff can't get to know patients in such a personal way. I know I, for one, have had my fair share of being on the other side and mostly treated with care, kindness and compassion by doctors and nurses. I have also had some bad times and, of course, like all things in life we have a ten-dency to remember the bad and forget the good. I think though that the irony as a doctor is that the bad experiences can positively influence the way a doctor treats patients thereafter.

I want to illustrate this for you with a few anecdotes, mostly medical but finishing with a non-medical personal story which was hugely ironic. I have three daughters who regularly accuse me of being an egotist, something I dearly hope I'm not, although most of us are guilty on occasion. When I was a newly qualified doctor, I worked in the Southern General Hospital in Glasgow, Scotland. This was my house job to allow me to develop some general medical skills, and well taught I was. Unfortunately, four months into the job, I and two colleagues went down with hepatitis. This was bad news; we were all very sick with high temperatures and severe sweats. My liver became swollen to twice its normal size and my spleen four times the norm. In addition, for the first three weeks, we had no idea of the cause. There was the further worry that we might have caught Hepatitis B. This is still not good but back then often fatal. This was the early eighties and, in the late seventies in Edinburgh Royal Infirmary, there had been an outbreak which had killed eight patients and four staff.

To further upset my apple cart a diagnosis of Hepatitis B or C would have been an end of my career dream of becoming a surgeon. There followed an unpleasant few weeks of feeling really unwell and thinking my career was over before it had started. I read *The Art of Advocacy* by Richard Du Cann reckoning that a legal career beckoned. I was looked after by three wonderful doctors, the late Dr Adams, Consultant Physician, Dr Alastair Starke, his Registrar, and Dr Bob Kilpatrick (sadly deceased), the senior SHO. They were three brilliant doctors, empathetic and knowledgeable. I also worked for them in my six months as their houseman. In that time I never saw Dr Adams make a wrong diagnosis, almost always based on the history and examination and sparse use of tests. He was in his sixties and I remember him telling me that we juniors always felt proud if we could think of over twenty tests to order when we had an emergency admission. In his day as a houseman, forty years earlier, they reckoned they were doing well if they produced five tests, mostly done by the doctor himself, not in the laboratory. He also, wisely, commented that forty years on I would find my juniors at the same stunt, but with even more tests He also wisely commented that there will always be patients who are diagnostic conundrums, we just don't know what's wrong with them; a very unsatisfactory place for a patient to find themselves. As our tests have got better the number of people in this position has greatly reduced, but has not vanished.

Two weeks into my sickness, I felt marginally better and bored being at home. I used to play tennis with Alastair Starke; I phoned him up to ask if he fancied a game. He was not impressed.

"You should be in hospital, not at home, we are managing you at home to make it easier for you. If you play tennis you will probably die from a ruptured spleen!"

That was me told. Just after this Dr Beatty, the liver specialist and also one of my bosses, had mooted the idea of a liver biopsy. Dr Adams asked me what I thought about the idea. The year before I had seen a poor man die from haemorrhage leading to a massive stroke following this procedure so I politely declined. He knew his patient and didn't push it. He said he quite understood and perhaps we would settle for an ultrasound—not a particularly effective diagnostic tool at that time. We both agreed. The following day I presented myself at the X-ray department as they were called then—now Imaging is the name to cover X-ray, MRI, CT, and ultrasound.

A typical Glasgow Auxiliary nurse, gruff but with a smile handed me a shopping basket, I was thinking I'm not here to go shopping, what's it for? She told me to enter into the horsebox like structure opposite, there were four in a row, take my clothes off and then go out the other side of the box into a waiting area. I stripped off down to my boxers and then leant out to ask if I should keep them on. I am a modest Scotsman. The reply? "I said all your clothes." I forgot to say she had also given me one of those ridiculous gowns that nobody knows which way round to wear; they have tapes for tying but if you put them on open at the front you expose yourself, the other way round your bare arse is on show if you are not careful. I went for closing at the back approach. I looked out one more time for advice.

"Do you want the shopping basket?"

"No, you keep your own clothes and go through the other door."

I step through the second door to find a waiting room full of people normally dressed, no silly gowns for them. Worse, they all started laughing at me. It's just as well I'm reasonably robust. I said to them," Do you want to know the best bit? I'm a doctor in this hospital."

At that they all howled with laughter, one of them said "Now you know how bad it is in this hospital!" At that, they all started clapping.

Now comes the icing on the cake, I'm called in for my scan by a complete dragon of a Consultant Radiologist. The room is dark, as scan rooms are. She doesn't even say hello, just "Get up on the couch and bare your tummy." I lift up my gown (opening at the back rather inconveniently at this point!) and she immediately says, "Why have you not got your underpants on? Get them on now! It's your liver I am scanning." She could easily have added "You perverted mollusc," but she didn't. I scrabbled about in the shopping basket to find them and then pulled them on. Task complete I had my scan which revealed a very large liver and spleen, already known about from being examined. What a waste of time and what humiliation but also many lessons learned about being a patient, worst being disempowered. To finish this story on a happy note, it transpired we had contracted toxoplasma hepatitis. As junior doctors, the high point of our day was a take-away meal in the evenings, at that time we worked eighty-four hours per week. That was seen as soft; up until 1980, the hours were often even longer. We all used to sit down together to eat; it transpired that we had been fed a dead cat in our Chinese take-away – big trouble for that takeaway, but thankfully the three of us recovered over a few weeks.

The lesson, I took from all of this was that good communication was key and that one's time as a patient is really scary, particularly if you don't know what is wrong with you or whether or not you're supposed to keep your pants on. So whatever is happening don't be afraid to ask your healthcare professional. You have every right to be treated with care and compassion.

A few years ago, I developed chest pain and took myself off to the Emergency Room of the Chelsea and Westminster Hospital. I was very effectively and promptly dealt with there. Then I was transferred up to coronary care unit. Loads of tests were done including a blood test called troponin. If this test is positive, you've had a heart attack, if not, you haven't. So many of our tests don't give straight answers. Biomedical tests don't work like straight mathematics. You will not like to hear what I am going to tell you but virtually every medical test ever performed has a built in false positive rate and false negative rate. In the false positive we tell you that there is a problem when there isn't, and in the false negative we tell you everything is okay when it isn't. Now it's obvious that the first leads to lots of anxiety, further tests and investigations but it plays safe. In the latter, it is plain dangerous, because of this all tests are slewed to false positivity, rightly, to maximise safety. Amongst my patients, people who deal with finance and accounting really hate this aspect of biomedicine; the physicists and mathematicians hate it the most.

I knew I could expect the result of a very reliable test at 6 a.m. the following morning and that, irrespective of the result, I was being transferred to the Royal Brompton for an angiogram. I woke about 5 a.m. and wondered what the result would be. Initially I had mixed feelings—sure, I didn't want to have had a heart attack but I also had a very expensive insurance policy which would have paid out massively if the test was positive. Of course, the closer 6 a.m. came the more I thought screw the money, please God let me not have had the heart attack. My prayers were answered and the test was negative. Later that morning, I was taken by ambulance to the Royal Brompton Hospital where I stayed for the next thirty hours. I so understand why patients don't want to be in hospital. I was starved from midnight before the procedure the following day. The angiogram was so skilfully performed and went well, and my heart was fine. I returned to the ward for a few hours of observation, much relieved but also starving hungry. This is a state I inflict on my patients too, although less so since what I am about to describe to you.

There was a really great nurse looking after me who had helped me order some food and said he would help me when it arrived. That may sound a bit soft but I had to lie horizontally for six hours to prevent a haematoma at the site where the wire had been inserted in my groin. Just before the food arrived, I could think of nothing else by this stage, two really sick patients were admitted and the nurse was really busy looking after them and they really needed him. The food arrived and was placed on a trolley at the bottom end of the bed. I could smell it and just see it, but of course quite rightly there was no nurse to help me eat it. I felt like a fraud, my coronary arteries were normal and the other two guys were sick, but, wow, my stomach was crying out for that food. I managed to get my foot under the trolley and bring it close enough to grab—remember I'm horizontal and have to stay that way. I then took the straw from my water and sucked up the soup. Adversity really is the mother of invention. I then spooned the main course across to my mouth with the plate lying on my chest, oh how wonderful to eat! The one thing I had not reckoned on was the inevitable need to burp having eaten in this way. I promise you, you cannot eat from a horizontal position and not need to burp and you can't burp from that position without vomiting, up

I sat and burped. Very satisfying. A small haematoma developed, I did not care.

I returned to work the following day, relieved at my good health and much more interested in how long I was starving my patients for. It's interesting because a lot of these things come under the category of suffering. This is a newly emerging field of study with measurable outcomes, very good news for all of us.

Saying sorry when we get it wrong can be one of the hardest things to do—in general and in the medical field. For years there was much confusion as to whether apologising when things had gone wrong was an admission of liability and therefore not advisable. There is now much more clarity around this and when things do go wrong there is "a duty of candour" placed on health care professionals that they should give a truthful explanation and that it is advisable to apologise. I think, possibly coming from a legal family, I took that position from early on. This partly came about from being caught out in my career.

I return to my houseman days at the Southern General Hospital. There was a man in his forties who I admitted to our ward as an emergency with shortness of breath. On his chest X-ray he clearly had a lot of fluid on one side of his chest, known as a pleural effusion. It was my job to insert a needle into his chest and suck some of this fluid out to send it for analysis. Also, removing the fluid would allow him to breathe more easily as an asthmatic, something I can easily empathise with. We had no idea what the fluid would reveal, perhaps an infection or, hopefully not, something more sinister. He remained in the ward and I got to know him well, he was a really good guy and we had a lot of laughing and joking. He had worked in the ship yards as a coker, somebody who cleaned out boilers. This occupation sadly led to his undoing. On the day the fluid analysis came back he did not have tuberculosis or any infection, but instead a dreaded mesothelioma of the lining of his lung. My Registrar asked me if I wanted to tell him the diagnosis or should he. I answered that I would. The Ward Sister looked at me and said "Are you sure you want to?"

"Yes I really am; I have got to know him well, I think it's my duty to." I had no idea what I was getting into. I approached him on the ward and sat down beside him. My face obviously said it all.

"You have bad news for me doctor?"

"Yes," I knew I must be truthful," I'm afraid you have a rare type of cancer in your chest."

"Is it lung cancer?"

"No, not the normal type, it's coming not from the lung but the lining of the lung. It's a mesothelioma." So far, so good, thinks I.

"Will it kill me doctor?" I hesitate and then reply "Yes, I'm afraid it will, I'm so sorry."

After a few moments, he says "How long have I got?"

"I don't really have any idea, to be honest." The first lie.

"You must have some idea, no?"

"Not really." Somehow comes out of my mouth, the second little economy of truth. My mind is whirring because the truth is too terrible; this is a disaster, this is a nasty cancer for which there were no treatments at that time, and back then it carried an average survival of 3 to 6 months. Then, as it still is now, it was associated with exposure to asbestos.

"Are we talking weeks, months or years?"

I then reply "Oh years, I hope." That was the whopper. The first two were evasions, the third was just plain wrong. I left him a few minutes later, to be followed by the Ward Sister visiting him. The first thing he said to her was "that Dr Smith's a decent fellow and he has told me what is wrong with me, and that it's bad, but he lied to me about how long I've got; I think it's much worse than he said." The Sister told him the truth.

She returned to the ward office and recounted her exchange. I felt terrible; I had lied not in any malicious way but lied nonetheless. I needed to apologise rapidly and returned shame-faced to say sorry. Easy to describe, bad to experience. I was no longer the smart young doctor I had seen myself to be.

However, mercifully, he was gracious, forgave my lie and we both agreed I had learned a valuable lesson. Truth is all and personal humility is vital.

The General Medical Council, the body which regulates doctors, rightly insists on a duty of candour and the need where appropriate to offer an apology. Over my whole career, like all doctors, things occasionally go wrong but most patients want three things: to know the truth; to receive an apology and to know what steps have been taken to prevent the same mistake being made with somebody else. Contrary to popular opinion the vast majority of wronged patients are not seeking money as the prime motivator for taking legal action. If we as professionals fail to deliver on the first three, they will and do take legal action and then money will often follow delivery of the truth and perhaps an apology. I would like to illustrate this to you with an example.

Most days one turns up in clinic and things run reasonably smoothly; there are, however, exceptions. The exceptions always seem to happen more often if you have an observer with you. I had been approached by a Senior Registrar in Sexually Transmitted Infections to sit in my gynaecology clinic as an observer. He would become a consultant within a year or two. Now I should point out that in medicine there is a bit of a divide between the physicians and surgeons. Traditionally, physicians felt it was the kiss of death to hand their patients over to the surgeons, certainly true until the twentieth century; some attitudes still prevail. The Senior Registrar in question was a physician and I could sense he arrived in my clinic with a healthy scepticism of my speciality. It is worth saying that one of the things which drew me to obstetrics and gynaecology was its mixture of medicine, surgery and psychology. It's also interesting that the Scottish tradition was much more towards medical gynaecology and obstetrics, with, in my day, trainees being encouraged to do a thesis or Membership of the Royal College of Physicians in addition to Membership of the Royal College of Obstetricians and Gynaecologists. The English tradition was much more towards gynaecological surgery with trainees encouraged to obtain Fellowship of the Royal College of Surgeons. This is reflected in titles; in Scotland gynaecologists are Dr, in England Mr or Mrs.

So, the two of us are sitting in Charing Cross hospital outpatient clinic and the nurse shows the first patient in. She sits down, making no eye contact. I know her well, I had performed her hysterectomy six weeks earlier.

"Are you Ok?" I said.

No response.

"Are you alright? Is something wrong?" She sat staring in front of her making no eye contact with me, or my colleague.

She finally replied, "I have entered a parallel universe since your op."

I had never heard that statement before, nor have I heard it since, thank goodness. A long consultation followed which did manage to get things back on track. My observer's adverse thinking about surgery and gynaecology was certainly getting some reinforcement.

Worse was to follow, the clinic, only just started was now running late. The second patient was shown in. I smiled, there was no smile back, and said hello, introduced my observer colleague.

"How are you?" I asked.

Her response went thus: "I am the victim of gross mismanagement by your hospital, I reckon you people have tried to cover it up, it's a total disgrace and I intend to sue you! Your people's mistakes have almost cost me my life."

This was truly awful. I normally carefully read the patient's notes before calling them in, but because I was running late, I had failed in this. As the woman was speaking, I suddenly realised who she was. She had indeed been mismanaged, badly. I, in fact, had chaired a prolonged meeting where we had investigated what had happened. We had identified two genuine mistakes which had led her to a bad place. We had changed our protocols as a result to prevent the same thing happening again. I had also requested the woman be brought back to see me to discuss her case. Her visit to the clinic was not as a result of this request, this was her "routine" follow up. In essence, she had an ectopic pregnancy which had been missed on two occasions with her being sent home twice from casualty when she should not have been—really not good—it was partly an issue about where we had drawn the line on a blood test level which was new at the time.

I took a deep breath and said to the patient, "I'm really sorry, I know exactly who you are and what has happened to you. I'm very sorry. We have had an enquiry about what happened to you and have made changes to how we manage ectopic pregnancies to stop this happening again. I have a proposal, I will take you through your notes page by page and explain to you where your management was good, OK, and wrong."

We duly did this over the next half hour. Understandably some of the things she felt were wrong were right and vice versa. At the end, she nodded.

"When I came in here I was going to sue you. I wanted the truth and to know that it won't happen again. I also wanted an apology for my suffering; I have had all three, thank you. You won't see me again, I'll be going to another hospital."

I apologised again and she left. My observer sat dumbfounded; I was chastened. I am forever grateful to that patient for her attitude, honesty and directness in the face of serious error; I personally felt very humbled by this experience. The remainder of that morning ran late but more like normal and over the course of the next year my observer and I got to a better place as well.

I want to finish this chapter with the interesting conundrum of when something goes wrong temporally close to a surgical procedure. Is it a surgical complication or just bad luck? I am going to tell you three stories here, each of which gives a different perspective.

A patient came to see me, she had bleeding between her periods. I organised an ultrasound scan for her which showed an endometrial polyp, I arranged for her admission for a hysteroscopy under a general anaesthetic. We saw said polyp, photographed it, removed it, photographed that it had gone and the cavity of the uterus had been made normal and then we sent the polyp for analysis. It was thankfully benign. The patient returned three months later with further bleeding between her periods, had an ultrasound and a polyp was seen. She attended my clinic and said, "Doctor, are you competent? Did you really remove the polyp?" Of course, here I had a watertight case, with photographic evidence and the pathologist's analysis confirming that I had removed a benign polyp. She apologised and I arranged to remove the new polyp. This was clearly a cut and dried scenario.

In the next scenario, I had a woman in the hospital who I had performed a hysterectomy on two days earlier. She started to pass large quantities of blood from her bottom. Both the patient and I were very worried that I had damaged her bowel, although I couldn't see how I could have, however she had never had this before and she had had a big operation forty-eight hours earlier. All very worrying, until she had a colonoscopy which revealed something completely coincidental and easily fixed. A colonic polyp was removed. Result, one relieved patient and surgeon.

My final example happened to me. In my late twenties, I had just moved to London from Glasgow. I went to the dentist. I had lost my middle front tooth some years earlier and an expensive Maryland bridge had been put in to fill the gap. These bridges were a porcelain tooth with titanium butterfly wings either side, allowing it to be bolted to the two adjoining teeth. My new London dentist peered into my mouth and said, "That's a pretty rough looking Glasgow Maryland bridge." He then took hold of said bridge, there was a nasty cracking noise, he said "f**k, eh, that was going to happen anyway." I looked down to see my three front teeth in his hand, I looked up to see him perspiring. "I don't think so" I retorted. "They have been in there for ten years."

Now who was right? In all probability, I was. Anyway, the big issue then was to sort it so I didn't leave his office looking like Count Dracula with a bad dentist. He did sort it with a very neat bridge of a different type. This involved taking the teeth on either side and putting posts through them, thus allowing a new bridge with three porcelain teeth to be fitted; very expensive, but I did get a good price. My parting shot was to ask "How long will the bridge last?"

"Ten to twenty years is the norm," came the reply.

I tell this story to illustrate when the balance of probability has moved, but it's still not for certain. Ten years later the new bridge felt as if it had become loose. I returned. I'm a Scotsman and not keen on going to the dentist for check- ups, maybe going every couple of years, or earlier if there is trouble. The bridge had been trouble free. Much looking and poking and prodding ensued at this visit and the bridge was declared in good order and then as a final check some jelly was applied. Unfortunately, bubbles appeared with moving the bridge; it was loose on one side. The dentist turned to me and said "We will just tap it and get it out."

I responded, "I don't like the sound of this tapping, it sounds like the use of a hammer. Could you break the bridge? How much is a new one?"

The dentist looked at me and replied "Yeah, I suppose it is a bit like a hammer and yeah, I could break it. It's £3000 for a new bridge. The question you have to ask yourself is, Is this your lucky day?"

That Clint Eastwood line that my generation just love to use—remember Steve earlier with the gun? I reflected very briefly and replied, "I don't think it is, I'll come back another day, when I do feel lucky."

He and his assistant laughed and I left. It was pre-Christmas and I needed to hold onto my money. Come the New Year, I felt lucky and returned. I sat in the chair. The dentist had a quick look, nothing had changed and he produced a device which gripped the bridge and then the tapper which, just as I had surmised, was a fancy chrome hammer. Multiple taps later and nothing was mov-ing. He asked for the wire, his assistant looked blank—that was very worrying, she had been there for years; the wire was clearly rarely used. He gesticulated to a cupboard and a piece of plastic coated wire appeared, I reckon it had come from the garden centre. It was green and the same size as you would use to tie up your roses. The wire was placed through under the gum and brought back out and twisted with a chromed flat-topped weight hanging off it, and this contraption was now hanging off my face. The tapper now really came into its own. The first tap was gentle, my head nodded all the same as the hammer hit the weight; no joy. The second and third taps got bigger and the movement of my head more severe. I appeared to have got into real head butting (also known as the Glasgow kiss) mode. It still failed to budge. I should say that the last two swings had been accompanied by the f-word; not from me, although I was thinking it.

My dentist and I were Celts so this word is popular and not offensive in the way it is often seen in the South East. With one last really big swing of the hammer, accompanied by "F**k it," the thing flew out across the floor. I sat up in the chair; was it my lucky day? Wow, it was. He gave it a wash and stuck it back in, it's still there twenty years later, or at least most of it.

The other important point I wish to illustrate with this story is that when things go wrong it isn't always somebody's fault. I knew my dentist was highly competent. The trouble is "things happen." The original tooth breakage didn't stop me returning over the years for the ongoing good quality treatment that I received. We live in a blame culture, but sometimes things "just happen".

Our Golden Rule in this chapter was "Doctors might be better doctors if they were patients themselves." All these anecdotes have, over the years, seemed to help my patients in their difficult circumstances. Healthcare professionals don't need to suffer too much from humility but a little is good for us! We have to remember we are only as good as our last case. As the patient you have the right to expect kind, caring and compassionate treatment.

Rule 9.

Don't frighten the patient. Healthcare professionals need to look the part and engage

Now this sounds pretty obvious and it should be, it's central to the general tenet of this book—hope and being frightened are not comfortable bedfellows. However, I want to touch on a few themes where this golden rule has been broken by me quite inadvertently.

In the early nineties I was a senior registrar in Watford working for Mr Victor Lewis. Victor was a great surgeon and surgical teacher; I know the way I perform a certain type of hysterectomy today is the way he taught me. He was also a man with many connections and through these we were graced with a series of supernumerary doctors. The first one to join us was a Dr Zarroug, who had come from the Middle East ; he was a splendid fellow who immediately fitted in to the department. He, within a few days, was joined by another supernumerary doctor also from the Middle

East. These two doctors got on well with the whole team. In the outpatient clinic they would sit either side of me during consultations. I always ask the patients if they mind having two doctors to observe the consultations and the vast majority of patients say yes; it is vitally important for teaching the next generation. A couple of weeks after these two doctors had become well ensconced we were sitting in clinic when the nursing Sister opened the door and announced, "Richard, we have another supernumerary." He duly flowed into the room, and I mean flowed, he was in full length white robes and had a white turban with a brass helmet under it and a spike sticking out the top. I looked up with a start and said, "Where have you come from?"

He replied "Heathrow."

I responded "Oh, OK, so where did you get *on* the plane?"

"Nigeria."

"OK," says I. "Not meaning to be rude but while I think your outfit very impressive I think it might scare the patients."

Zarroug immediately got up and said he would take him shopping. The following day he reappeared dressed in a pinstripe suit; he had joined the team.

There is a serious point to be made here which relates to cross-cultural issues. Patients tend to want to be treated by doctors in their own country, there are plenty of French patients heading from London to Paris for healthcare and vice versa with the British, but it also runs to how the doctor is dressed. In London, consultant gynaecologists are always expected to wear suits. In clinic, jacket should be off with either a short-sleeved shirt or sleeves rolled up so as to be bare below the elbow. White coats have gone and scrub suits are not popular, more on this in a minute, ties are only allowed if tucked into a waistcoat, hence most men now have open necked shirts. Contrast this to Scandinavia where all medical staff in out-patients are in uniforms. Our dress code so upsets Scandinavian patients that they will often comment on British lack of cleanliness—not true but their perception. Funnily enough when it comes to scrub suits one of my colleagues, Mr Roger Marwood, had banned his juniors from wearing scrub suits in case they frightened the patients; I have to confess to being a little cynical as to whether this really was the case. He was right, as I discovered, when I appeared in my own clinic in a scrub suit. Fifteen minutes into the first consultation I suggested to the patient that she needed an operation and she looked appalled. I said, "I'm sorry I don't mean to frighten you but why do look so scared?" She looked at me and said "Do you want to operate on me right now?" I replied, "No, of course not, sometime in the next few weeks at a time to suit you." She then pointed at my scrub suit and said, "I thought you had come looking for people to operate on!" Wow, talk about giving the wrong impression!

As a student, I inadvertently upset a patient when we were having bedside teaching. I was in fourth year, my second clinical year. I had turned up on Professor Sir Abraham Goldberg's teaching ward round. Professor Goldberg was the world expert on a rare blood disorder called porphyria. That particular morning, I have to confess I was badly hung over and was paying no attention to the teaching whatsoever when Professor Goldberg asked the question "what is myosis?" I had my head down and had not realised that the professor was addressing the question to me. I realised I was in trouble when he tapped my shoulder. I had to ask that the question be repeated. It duly was and I replied, "!t is the process of gamete reduction during spermatogenesis." This got the response, "You stupid boy, we are looking at the patient's eyes." The poor patient moved from concern to amusement as he realised what a fool of a student he was dealing with.

To explain, myosis/miosis is excessive constriction of the pupil in the eye, meiosis (pronounced the same way) is where the ovaries and testicles reduce the chromosomes from 46 to 23 thus allowing reproduction when sperm meets an egg and the newly formed conceptus obtains 23 chromosomes from the female and 23 from the male adding up to the 46 chromosomes we all have. This was not my finest moment that's for sure, but no long-term harm was done.

We live in an age of increasingly casual dress, but healthcare professionals do vitally important things to patients and we need to remember our appearance and engagement are vital parts of the experience.

Rule 10.

A cup half empty can become a cup half full

DABDAH and the Landscape of Grief

DABDAH, is the acronym for the range of emotions associated with the grief response. D stands for denial, A for anger, B for bewilderment and bargaining—are these results really mine? Could there be a mistake? The second D is for depression and then comes A for acceptance and H for hope. These were originally described, although not including H for hope by Dr Elizabeth Kubla-Ross in the 1950s. They came to be seen, by many, as a linear process, although that is not implicit in her treatise.

This concept has evolved into the pictorial model 'the landscape of grief.' This is Fr Gary Bradley, Vicar of Little Venice's construct. He is Chairman and founder of the Westminster Bereavement Association and has developed this model to help explain the grieving process. I regularly use this model with patients. The analogy I draw is that most of us have pictures on the wall at home. I accept there are a few minimalists with none! However, assuming you are not one of this group, you have pictures on the walls. When you purchased them, something drew you to them out of the other pictures in the gallery or shop. After you had made the purchase you took the picture home and hung it up. For the first few weeks thereafter, you would look at the picture and see the same thing but as time went by, if the picture is any good, you will see new things appear that you hadn't noticed originally. This is much more how the emotions come and go. This is much more like Fr Gary's landscape of grief. This again is fully described in my books *Women's Cancers: Pathways to Healing* and *Women's Cancers: Pathways to Living*.

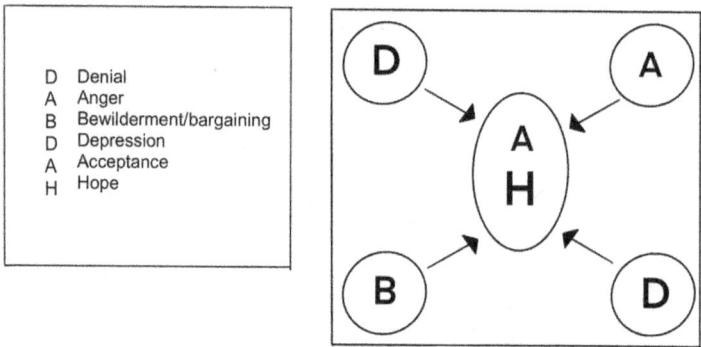

D	Denial
A	Anger
B	Bewilderment/bargaining
D	Depression
A	Acceptance
H	Hope

Fig 8. DABDAH and the landscape of grief

Of course, issues with respect to fertility are heavily wrapped up in this process—loss of fertility compounding depression, maintenance of it speeding the path to acceptance and hope.

There is one further pictorial model I have seen and used which was developed by Dr Nicola Holton, a palliative care specialist in Norwich. If a patient gets stuck at the bottom of the loop, they think they can't get out. What follows are strategies to help those people.

Change: The Transition Curve

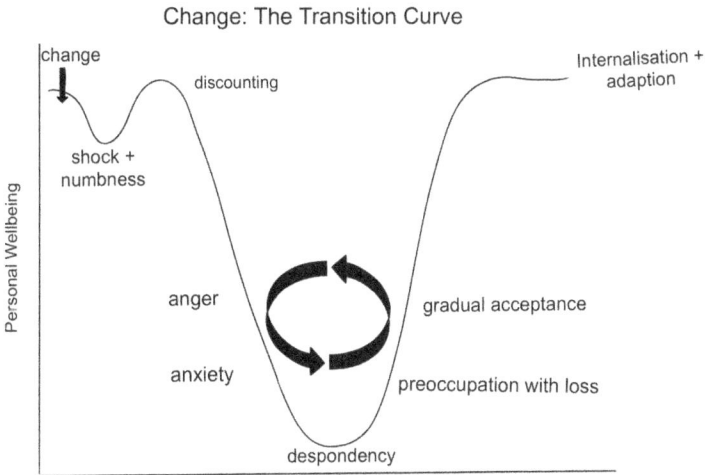

Fig 9: The grieving process, by Dr Nicola Holton

The next pictorial model for patients on the cancer pathway is the following Venn Diagram.

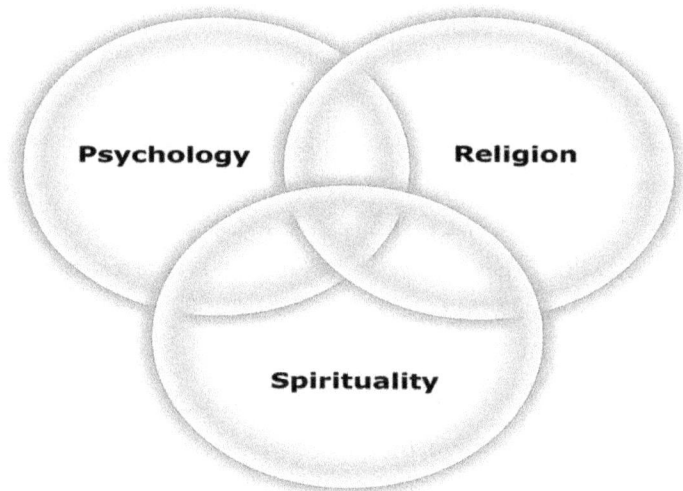

I will tend to slide a hand-drawn version of this across the table when the patient is four to six weeks post-surgery and may be about to start chemotherapy. I am careful to point out that I am not out to proselytise for any particular religion or indeed any religion at all. It surprises many patients and their relatives but the commonest time for the patient to go on a real downer is at the end of treatment when physical recovery is complete or close at hand. This Venn diagram allows further all-encompassing discussion to take place. It allows the politically sensitive subject of religion to be brought in which again, in the cancer and fertility setting, can be vitally important.

Spirituality is also important to some/many and there is no doubt in my mind if we are aiming for a truly holistic approach to our patients, then where appropriate this subject needs to be broached. One of the difficulties here is that Priests tend to shy away from psychology, psychologists shy away from religion and spirituality. Doctors and nurses are rightly wary of discussing the latter two and the patient may fall through the middle where discussion takes place at all. One of the few writers who crosses these boundaries is the great Swiss psychologist Carl Gustav Jung, whose works such as *Man in Search of a Soul* delve into this area. Jung was fascinated by dreams, "the dream is the little hidden door in the innermost and most secret recesses of the psyche..." He coined the term individuation which is that stage in life usually in our late 30s or around 40 years of age when we finally stop trying to get a response from our parents. We are as we are. This can also be a significant factor when caring for the young woman with cancer. Jung believed in the collective sub-conscious, and coined the term synchronicity whereby things happen to us way beyond what should happen by chance. A new term for this is morphic resonance and readers who are interested should explore Rupert Sheldrake's writings and lectures. Jung was convinced that all of us have to address these issues for our psychological well-being. What conclusion we each come to doesn't matter, it's the fact we have addressed it.

Many years ago, I lectured to the Charing Cross Cancer Patients Association on the subject of Doctor-Patient communication. There were fifty-five people, mainly women, who all had or had had cancer. This was definitely Daniel entering the lion's den, what in Glasgow (my home town) would be regarded as a bit of a punt! There was a flip chart and no other audio-visual props. I talked them through the four cusps, then DABDAH and the Landscape of Grief and then onto the Venn diagram. However, that evening I decided to expand a little. I said to the audience, who had been polite and attentive until that point, that I wished to cause no offence and if I did, I apologised in advance, but asked if they would indulge me for the next ten minutes while I discussed spirituality and religion.

The response was amazing, the quiet audience erupted. One woman shouted "this is what we want to talk about," another shouted "You and your bloody nurses won't talk to us about this, it's the most important thing!"

So how have we ended up in a situation where doctors and nurses run in fear of their livelihood if they discuss this subject, but in the process are letting many people down badly? It is clearly very important that doctors and nurses should never proselytise for their own religion, but we should be able to at least discuss these issues.

That evening for me proved pivotal and certainly emboldened me to lecture and teach more on this. I explore these issues in more depth in another of my books *The Journey: Spirituality, Pilgrimage and Chant*.

We have discussed earlier the four cusps for those in cusps A and B, in other words those who are free of disease, 'cured' or 'living with cancer,' these are the majority of patients in my practice. There seems to me to be an almost bimodal distribution of patient response, what I would call the cup half full versus the cup half empty brigade.

Most things in nature follow a standard distribution curve. An example would be to look at the age a woman will go through the menopause. The range considered normal is between 40 and 56—below the age of 40 years is abnormally early, as over the age of 56 years is abnormally late—the average age is 51 years old. This statement is based on a standard distribution curve. 95% of values lie within two standard deviations of the mean, 99.7% within three standard deviations.

In terms of cancer diagnosis, one group of patients following treatment lapse into long-term fear of recurrence, thus spoiling the time they have in remission. Remember that however good a prognosis the tumour one has may recur and, likewise for the patient with a poor prognosis tumour, sometimes things turn lucky and they beat the statistics. This is why survival statistics are great for comparing treatment modalities, but for the individual patient not very helpful. To illustrate this, I will give you two examples. A 51-year-old woman comes to me with an endometrial cancer. She has her uterus, Fallopian tubes and ovaries removed and proves to have a Grade 1 (tumours are graded 1, 2, 3; 1 being best, 3 worst), Stage 1a endometrial cancer. This is one of the best prognosis cancers we see, and carries a 98% 5-year survival. Sadly, nine months later she develops secondary cancer in her lungs and dies rapidly—the good statistics were meaningless to the individual patient. In contrast, many years ago now a patient was admitted to the Chelsea and Westminster in a very sick way with a disseminated ovarian cancer which had spread to her chest (Stage IV). She very unusually asked me not how long she had to live: "what are my 5-year survival statistics?" In patients with gynaecological cancers, survival at 5 years without having had a recurrence in that 5 years is usually but not always associated with cure—the cured circle aimed for in Cusps A and B that we discussed earlier. This is sadly not the case in some breast cancers which can return after many years in remission. I told my patient that she had a 25% five years survival but, such was the nature of her disease, that cure lay at less than 5%. Today this 25% has become 50% in the best centres but the cure rate has not improved so much. This patient then underwent chemotherapy followed by surgery. At the time of her surgery I removed her uterus, Fallopian tubes, ovaries, omentum and para aortic and pelvic lymph nodes. For the record the omentum is a fatty thing hanging off the large bowel and stomach in all of us; it gets called the abdominal policeman, because it goes to where there is trouble. Unfortunately, in cancers, this is unhelpful since the omentum is a common place for ovary cancers to spread to. In this patient's case, while there was tumour in most things removed the three pulses treatment of chemotherapy had killed the whole cancer except for a few viable cells in one para aortic lymph node. She had a further three pulses of chemotherapy and has since passed both the 5 and 10-year marks in complete remission and returns yearly to give me a hug. This demonstrates our first golden rule, never say never. There is an irony because aggressive grade 3 tumours are often more chemo-sensitive, as proved in this case. This patient went on to become a seriously cup-half-full individual, adopting many strategies to gain control of her life again.

Having, I hope, demonstrated the uncertainty involved with any cancer prognosis, I now want to return to the theme of the cup-half-full brigade versus the cup-half-empties. The cup-half-full people often perceive that their cancer diagnosis, far from being a negative thing, has helped them into a new mind set where they live every day to the full. They have discovered how to be in the moment. Meanwhile, the cup-half-empties live in fear of recurrence and all the other deep-seated fears we humans have—this can often run for years, having a terrible effect on their and their family's quality of life.

This either or attitude also applies to the women with HIV and, of course, the women who cannot conceive. These are all scenarios where women are dealing with uncertainty which may go on for years or even be lifelong.

To me, one of the big challenges is how to turn the cup-half-empties into half fulls. This issue becomes all the more important as survival figures improve, many more patients discovering that after 5 years they are cured. Those who are not cured but are in remission between courses of treatment need to have strategies for living in the moment.

My books, *Pathways to Living* and *The Journey; Spirituality, Pilgrimage, Chant* describe methods of self-help including taking control of one's diet, learning self-hypnosis, walking with a pedometer and chant either performed in a religious repetitive prayer mantra or via heart math, which is a secular form of chant. I intend to explore these a little more here.

To quote Maggie Keswick Jencks, co-founder of Maggie's Cancer Caring Centres, "Above all, what matters is not to lose the joy of living for the fear of dying," or, as Buddha put it, "we need to develop the art of living rather than the fear of dying."

Much of what is required relates to people with cancer regaining control. This is where exercise, nutrition, chant and self-hypnosis can all come into. While chant and hypnosis bring one to a similar place, I am personally quite convinced they are not the same place. I was originally taught hypnotherapy in 1983 in Stobhill Hospital in Glasgow. I have been very fortunate in life with the friends I have made. I turned up as a new Senior House Officer in 1983 and met my new Registrar, Sam Abdalla, who had arrived from Baghdad. In amongst our many duties within obstetrics and gynaecology, Sam was taught how to hypnotise patients by Dr Giles, the oldest of the consultant group, he then taught me.

There used to be tutorials where about fifteen doctors gathered once a week. Sam decided to give a tutorial on hypnotherapy and, for demonstration purposes, I was to be his subject. He hypnotised me by a technique which I will expand on a little later. He then told me that the number 5 did not exist. He asked me to count to 10. I confidently counted 1, 2, 3, 4, 6, 7, 8, 9, 10, missing the number 5 but with no realisation of this. He then asked me what 2 and 4 was? I answered 6, then 2 and 3 and of course I did not know the answer because the number 5 had gone from my mind. I found this disturbing. He then gave me the number 5 back again and my arithmetic returned to normal. Much more powerfully he then asked me to cannulate my own vein on the back of my hand. This I duly did and of course blood started to flow from the cannula. He told me to stop bleeding, I did. Then he told me to restart bleeding, I duly did, finally I was told to remove the cannula, and I obliged. The group of doctors, by this time, were on the edge of their seats. It was clear to all that this technique had huge medical applicability.

One of the great difficulties for hypnosis in Glasgow at that time was a show in the Pavilion theatre with a stage hypnotist called Robert Halpern. Our year, in either the fourth or final year of university, went as a group to see him in action. He first used a simple technique to ascertain who was susceptible, namely he told the audience to clasp their hands together and he then told us that as he counted to ten our hands would get tighter and tighter. I now know I am very susceptible to hypnosis but I didn't then. My hands started to get tighter, but I had no desire to get on Halpern's stage, so I let them go. About fifty people ended up on his stage—I think this must represent some conscious or subconscious desire to be on the stage. Of the fifty he rapidly assessed the best subjects and used them for the rest of the show. At the end, he hypnotised himself and then hung himself on a rope, but survived. Not one to try at home! This was all highly entertaining but not a good advert for therapeutic hypnotherapy. Now, the even bigger problem was that this show attracted up to

1500 people a night, three nights a week—he was hugely popular and most of Glasgow had seen him in action. Everybody, therefore, had gained a very firm impression that hypnosis allowed the hypnotiser enormous control over their subject. In medical terms this is not the case. I'm sure that Halpern's technique selected the few exhibitionists in the audience while the rest of us kept clear of his stage.

The theory behind hypnotherapy is encapsulated in the drawing below.

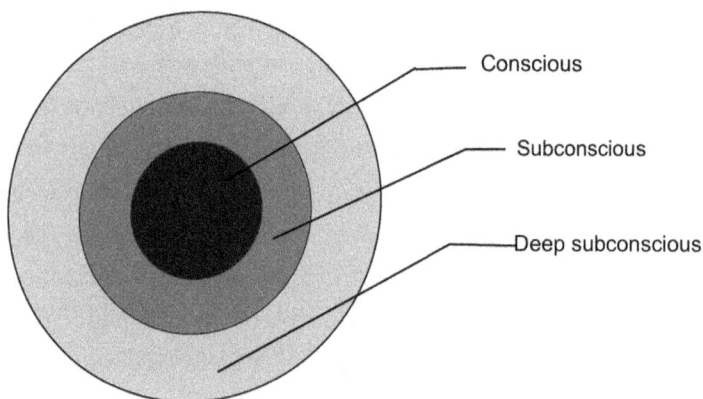

Fig 11

Normally we only have access to our conscious mind, however there are things going on in our subconscious and deep subconscious all the time, most of which we cannot get to. With respect to the subconscious, dreams are one of those hidden doors into this area. For the deep subconscious, an example would be one's heart rate. You can feel your pulse but you cannot will it to rise or fall. In a trance-like state you can tell yourself, or be told, that the pulse will rise or fall and it does. Breathing would be another example—normally you never think about, but if I asked you to hold your breath, you can, at least for a while. Thus, the conscious can sometimes influence the deep subconscious, but in general the subconscious and deep subconscious are difficult to access. However, in hypnotherapy, one can gain access to both the subconscious and deep subconscious and use this for therapeutic purposes.

There is much new thinking about pain management. If you have a pain in your right index finger there is the stimulant at the finger, the pathway to your spinal cord, the spinal cord pathway to your brain and then your brain's appreciation of the pain. In pain management terms, you can sort out the stimulant at your finger e.g. remove the stimulant or take an anti-inflammatory. You can interrupt the pathway to your spinal cord, e.g. inject local anaesthetic into the digital nerve and the finger goes numb, or insert a spinal cord neuromodulator (very expensive) and moderate the pain or you can try to act on the brain by use of drugs (both painkillers and centrally acting antidepressants but not used in antidepressant doses). Finally, you can try techniques such as hypnotherapy which work with the brain's plasticity. Remember, at the end of the day all pain is felt in the brain. That does not mean it is imaginary as patients sometimes think. This is very important and I will hear medical students say, "Oh the pain is in the patient's head." This is almost invariably not true. The patient with pain who is properly investigated usually will have a diagnosis made, however the treatment may involve moderating that pain at 'the head end.'

I use the technique which Sam taught me to hypnotise patients and myself. These days, unfortunately, I do not have enough time to hypnotise anybody apart from myself and two of my four children—two are susceptible and two think it is rubbish. The one exception to this being during Covid 19 lockdown when I was asked by the Sylvan Retreat Centre of North London to do an on line Zoom entitled Hypnosis for sleep. I was somewhat apprehensive but agreed to do it. I found myself hypnotizing ninety people on line but it was well received and they asked me to do it again for YouTube. If you are interested it is entitled Self Hypnosis for sleep: https://youtu.be/q6oplS4kXvs. For the last twenty plus years I have referred patients to my colleague Shaun Hammond. I have been hypnotised by him many times and his techniques are similar to my own although much more advanced.

In terms of who makes a good candidate, the answer is most people. In contrast to what people usually think, to be a good candidate you do not to be weak willed. In fact, the principle guiding factor is the ability to concentrate and not let the mind wander. Strong personalities are often good at this. Cynicism also tends to increase with age and this can be a complete block to success.

The question many people ask is what does it feel like? This is quite hard to answer, but while one is completely aware one is also removed. It feels pleasant, in fact sometimes so pleasant that one doesn't want to wake up. It is not the same but shares some properties with how one might feel after taking a sleeping tablet or a mildly hallucinogenic drug.

Now how does one go about this? Firstly, I ask you to lie on a couch or sit in a relaxing reclining chair. I could use a Halpern style susceptibility test of hand clasping or telling you your head feels heavy and watching for you to start nodding. I don't however do this. Instead, I start with some breathing exercises. I ask you to breathe in through your nose, unless you are a mouth breather. I then ask you to breathe out through your mouth to the count of ten, and to imagine you are blowing a candle out. After a few minutes of this, I ask you to tense your toe muscles and let them relax, tense your calf muscles and let them relax, tense your thighs and let them relax. You will feel yourself sinking into the couch. Then tense your tummy muscles and let them relax, then shrug your shoulders and relax, then screw up your face and relax. By now you will be feeling really good and I ask you to tip your head back. I stand or sit slightly behind you and ask you concentrate on the tip of my pen which I hold slightly above and behind your eyes so they are under slight strain to see it. I then tell you I am going to count to ten and your eyelids will feel heavier and heavier. I count to ten, your eyelids start to flicker and I suggest that you should give way to the heavy feeling and close them. You close your eyes and feel beautifully relaxed. I now ask you to imagine you are either on the beach and about to walk down into the water or on a heather-clad hillside with a brook at the bottom and you are about to descend. In either case, you can feel a breeze, it's bright and sunny and you can hear the water. If you are on the beach you can smell the sea, if you are on the hillside, you can smell the heather. As you can see, all of your senses are stimulated, sight, feel, smell and sound. I then tell you I am going to count from one to ten and you will either walk down the beach or descend the hill and as you do so you will go deeper and deeper into sleep. This process can then be repeated to get even deeper.

Once you have arrived in the deep trance state, I will be able to see that you are breathing through your tummy and not your chest. We will together do the therapeutic part of the treatment which I will illustrate later with some personal examples. I then tell you that the next time you come back you can go down into your trance by counting from one to five on the tips of your fingers. You brush your thumb against the index finger, then the middle one, then the ring finger then your little finger and then back to your index finger. This means that, in contrast to the first consultation which will take about an hour, the subsequent one takes thirty minutes. You will also be able to use this technique to hypnotise yourself.

I then tell you that you will never be hypnotisable ever again except by a doctor, dentist, psychologist or someone that you know and trust including yourself. This protects you in future from the likes of Halpern. I then wake you up by counting back from five to one and you wake up slowly feeling very relaxed and at one with yourself. You may be resistant to waking up because the feeling is good, but you will. Everybody does and I will have told you this before we started to alleviate any anxieties on this front.

I have been hypnotised many times but I will give you two personal examples which may be helpful to demonstrate the power of the technique. Many years ago, when I was in my late twenties, I went to Shaun Hammond to stop smoking cigarettes and to lose weight. At the time, I was smoking twenty cigarettes per day and was two stone overweight. I am also asthmatic. Shaun hypnotised me and once I was in a trance he used a Buddhist/Hindu concept. He asked me which of my chakras I thought was strongest—head, face, heart, gut or groin. For me the strongest place is my chest. As you know we all often describe people as head strong, big heart, or driven by their groin! For me it's the heart. I was then asked to imagine my chest opening up like flower. Once open it was bathed in pure light and my dirty asthmatic lungs washed with water. After this I was asked to let the power in my chest flow out of it like a fountain. Once I could feel this I was asked to close the flower down and feel the power instead coursing to my fingertips.

Following this I was asked to describe where I most liked to smoke. I described the terrace in front of my family's house on Bute, one of the islands off the west coast of Scotland. From there I was taken to a room, my "Room 101". In it there was a television and a door. I was in the television and in the room synchronously. The me in the TV was me twenty years later. I had developed chronic bronchitis and could only breathe assisted with an oxygen mask and I suffered terrible coughing fits. Shaun gave me a choice, either to be in the television, or in the room with the television and the door. I could walk through the door which had just opened. On the other side was the fresh air and sunshine of Bute and being a non-smoker. I started to walk to the door but hesitated. Shaun asked me what I wanted to do. Be in the

"Room 101" as a smoker or in the fresh air as a non-smoker? This time I walked through the door and haven't smoked again in well over two decades. I gained no weight, in fact I lost the two stone. It proved easy to say no to cigarettes and food. Every time I felt the urge I would self-hypnotise and, using the power of the chest chakra going down to my fingertips, I would psychologically push the offending item away.

I do quite a lot of lecturing and public speaking to students, doctors, patient groups and others. There are few who do not feel nervous prior to these events, particularly with big audiences. It is ironic, however, that it usually proves easier with a bigger audience than a small one. In a large auditorium, the people in audience themselves are nervous to speak out and you already hold the floor making it harder for the audience to give you a bad time. However, you never know how it will go until you've done your talk. At the end of the day public speaking is like surgery – you are only as good as your last speech or operation. Before all big talks, I will be sitting in a self-induced trance in the run up to the speech. I then imagine the chest chakra and feel that power flowing though me. I then count back from five to one, "wake up" and can walk to the podium feeling relaxed and confident.

In terms of hypnotism as a form of pain-management, I had a patient who was suffering from vulval pain, a very distressing symptom. This particular case was part of my deciding that, in general, I was better to refer to Shaun. She had been fully investigated by way of excluding infection, pre-cancer skin conditions and any specific neuroma formation, etc. I hypnotised her using the techniques described above. Having obtained a deep trance. I told her that her pain was flowing down her legs and through her feet and then out of her toes in fountains; this is a standard technique. I then woke her up and asked her how she was. She said she was pain free for the first time in years. Amazing. I asked her to return in a week to check her progress which she duly did. She walked in with a limp and wearing over size trainers, before trainers were even trendy. I asked about her vulval pain, it had gone. Very good.

I asked, "What is wrong with your feet?"

To my horror she replied, "I don't know. When I went home last week I had this terrible pain in my feet,"

"What did it feel like?" I interjected.

"Oh, just like the pain I used to have in my nou nou."

This was bad. "Can I see your feet, please? What have you done to help the pain?" says I.

"I burnt my shoes" and at this point she took off her trainers and socks off to reveal toes wrapped in cotton wool. Worse still she had no insight into the hypnosis doing this. I was frightened. The next thing would be she was referred to a foot specialist who would find nothing wrong and presume her mad or her gynaecologist some sort of cowboy. I decided there and then to re-hypnotise her and put the pain back where it had started, namely in her vulva. I duly did this and to my relief the pain returned to its original site. I then called a friend; Shaun. He informed me that the fact that I had moved the pain from the vulva meant the strategy was right and I should have persevered. I decided not just to phone a friend, it was time to refer to a friend. Shaun rendered her pain free. I often recount this anecdote to patients who I am referring for hypnotherapy.

Just before we leave pain management I can't help but tell you a wonderful anecdote. There was a middle-aged woman who had a chronic pain at the top of her vagina for months; this is much rarer than pain at the entrance. She had, over time, had many investigations and treatments with no success. This particular afternoon she walked in with her partner, He was a professional engineer. They both smiled and I returned their smile. The boyfriend then said, "I'm an engineer and I've cracked it where you failed."

The patient smiled and I said, "Really, the pain has gone?"

'Yes," she said.

"You have to tell me how." I had tried every trick I knew.

"Listen." They went quiet, as did I. There was a faint buzzing noise. He said, "Do you hear that? That's a vibrator."

At that we all laughed. I asked if there were any issues, apart from the noise. There was one, it kept slipping when she walked about. At this point I could offer something.

"You should go down to John Bell & Croydon, Britain's biggest pharmacy, and get them to make you a belt to hold it in." I have never seen this patient again and hope she is still smiling.

This led me on to trying this 'vibration treatment' in another patient. It is not illogical to think it might work—physiotherapists use vibration therapy over damaged joints. I had this treatment on my knee years ago after a skiing injury. The patient in question attended clinic in the Chelsea and Westminster with an almost identical story. She was elderly and lived alone. I thought, well, somehow I have to bring this in to the conversation, but how? I then recounted the story I have told you above but immediately followed it up by asking if she had a partner—no she did not. I then said the difficulty was how she was going to get a vibrator, since this was before the days of internet ordering. I said, "I'm not being sleazy but they are only purchasable from sex shops. I don't guess that's the kind of place you go?" She looked at me as if I were deranged. I had a nurse with me, so I had a witness that I wasn't being inappropriate. "The problem is I can't prescribe it, they have to be bought."

She looked embarrassed, so I quickly offered to get my research fellow to purchase one, and told her we would send it to her in the post. I duly dictated a letter to the Fellow asking that he do this. There was much amusement in the secretaries' office over this letter. He, in fact, came back to me saying he didn't know any sex shops so I was left to purchase it myself—it was called The Lady's Finger and cost £10 with batteries. I may say I am not a big one for sex shops myself, but there were loads round Leicester Square; a bit seedy, I'll grant you. I sent it to the patient but never heard from her ever again. So, in a short trial of two at that time we had one success and one "lost to follow up."

We are now going to turn from vibrators to the slightly more obscure subject of repetitive prayer, or chant, and I hope to demonstrate the albeit subtle difference with the trance like state I have just described to you. Chant, I believe, takes one to a different place from hypnotic trance. I think hypnotherapy is great for 'rebooting' the brain when one's emotions are getting it wrong. We all go through times when the logical part of our brain knows we don't have a problem but our emotions are not giving us the same message. Hypnosis will work really well here, if the subject is susceptible.

However, to get us living in the here and now, chant is far better. All the world's prominent religions have sects who chant— Christian, Jewish, Sufi, Muslim, Hindu and of course those who follow the Buddha. In the Orthodox Christian and Jewish faiths this is called the Prayer of the Heart. In the Eastern religions, a mantra. The mere fact that I have used chant, repetitive prayer and mantra interchangeably suggests they are tapping into the same thing. I am not qualified to comment but the technique of mindfulness seems to be a secular approach to the same issues.

Returning to the secular approach, one of my colleagues Dr Tony Yardley-Jones, Consultant in Occupational Health, has been working with a new technique called cardiac coherence. This measures heart rate variability and the pictures below show the pattern when we are agitated and when we have a special reflective moment, by that I mean the feeling we get when we see a beautiful sunset or listen to certain pieces of music.

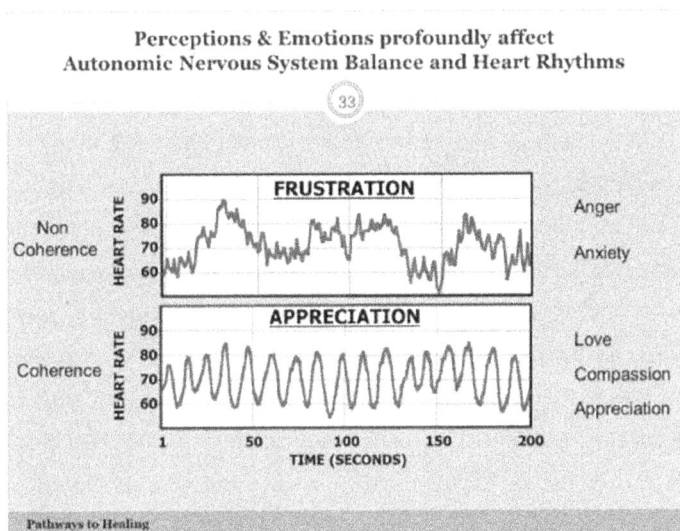

Fig 12

The jagged line gives way to a sinusoidal wave pattern. If you learn chant you achieve the same technique. When one's heart is in the sinusoidal pattern a feeling of appreciation and well-being runs strongly in one. Currently there is quite a lot of research looking at singing and well-being, including choirs specialising in chant. There is a bunch of London city bankers who are apparently right into it! Tony certainly put me to the test after hearing Shaun and I talk about trance versus chant. He appeared in my office at the end of a very busy clinical day with his device which he placed on my finger. At the end of the day I had always worried it was all in my head, but it isn't, it's in my heart too! The trace started all jagged, just what you would expect in the office, but within a minute of the mantra I had gone to the sinusoidal trace and felt good with myself.

This chapter I hope has demonstrated there are many approaches to transitioning from cup half empty to cup half full. These are all strategies to live in the now. Different approaches suit different people, the important thing is to grasp the issue. So much of this is about strategies to live "in the moment of now." Feroze Dada, of the Sylvan Retreat Centre, as part of a series of documentary interviews, interviewed me for Apex TV and explores the ideas of this chapter. It is entitled *Our One World* – Dr Richard Smith – A Healer's Vision. This was done in support of Womb Transplant UK Charity.

Rule 11.

Walk the walk, swim the swim and chant the chant

Exercise is extremely important in the cancer patient taking hold of their own destiny. Walking and swimming are two things most of us can do and they are cheap. There is nothing wrong with gym-based exercise if you like it. I don't. Running is fine but bad for your joints, walking to my mind is where it is at. So is swimming, although it is great cardiovascular exercise it is no use for bone density maintenance. That is where walking comes in.

Many years ago, I heard Michael Stroud lecture. He is the doctor who walked across Antarctica with Ranulph Fiennes— now that's what you call a walk! His hypothesis was that if you purchase a pedometer and make sure you are doing 10,000 steps in total, three days per week as a minimum, you would improve your bone density without drugs. Since then I have advised many osteopenic patients (where there is a trend towards thinning of the bones) to do this to great effect. I will advise those with osteoporosis (thin bones at risk of fracture) to see a rheumatologist and then a combination of drugs and exercise can be prescribed. These may include hormone replacement therapy (HRT), much maligned and until recently much underused. HRT may also be important to maintain the uterus in a reproductive state when the ovaries have been removed for cancer management and the patient is considering a donated egg pregnancy.

In terms of bone density, when you check it by a low dose X-ray there are only three results. It is either normal, it shows osteopenia—a trend in the direction of osteoporosis—or it shows osteoporosis itself. This means that one is at risk of fracture either at the wrist, hip, or lumbar vertebra. Women, on average, after the menopause, will lose half their bone mass within twenty years. This is very important since the average age for the menopause is 50-51 years (Range of normal 40-56 years) and the average life expectancy in the UK for a woman is around 85 years. Thus, many women may be at risk of fracture for many years. Data relating to the menopause and fertility will be discussed in more detail later. The reality is, if you walk you don't get osteoporosis and it can be screened for. It is, in other words, a totally preventable condition. It was considered by the UK National Screening Committee, but rejected on the grounds of cost. This is to do with health economics—the older you get the less valuable you are to the economy and this is put into the equation and so there is no national screening programme, but the test is available on request. This is understandable, particularly in the current economic climate, but I urge you to spread the word.

So, what is 10,000 steps, I hear you say? In one hit it is, approximately, a five-mile walk. I know for me, in an average working day, I will walk about one to two miles and I therefore need to do three to four miles more extra on top of this. If you want to find out what you are doing, buy a pedometer or consult the app on your smartphone or, if you are feeling very extravagant buy a Fitbit or Apple watch.

At the end of Michael Stroud's lecture, I went to congratulate him and bought his book. He didn't seem too bothered by my congratulations, but the book did change my life. I went and bought a pedometer expecting to readily hit the target, because I went for long walks at weekends and stood around in the operating theatre for hours but, as it transpired, I literally stood around.

When I bought the device, I found I got to way beyond on weekends (15,000-25,000 steps) but mid-week, as described above, nowhere close. I radically changed my week's structure with respect to commuting and started to walk to and from work on one to two days, and if I was going out in the evening I would walk to and from the venue. I rapidly found I was fitter, it did not eat into my working day, I spent less on petrol and I became addicted to the pedometer. Thank you to Michael Stroud.

Swimming is of no use for bone mineral density, it is however wonderful cardiovascular exercise. Cold water swimming may well have added benefits. There is good evidence for boosted immunity, enhanced circulation, and increased libido. The old saying of "Go take a cold shower!" in fact has the opposite effect. In addition, you burn more calories in cold water rather than warm water swimming. Recently, Wim Hof has sprung to fame producing much evidence to back up these ideas.

Both swimming and walking increase the production of the body's own opiates—endorphins. These have a serious feel-good factor and, like all opiates, are addictive. It's why people who take exercise can't stop. I know I have an element of bias and all exercise is good, but the great thing about swimming and walking is that you are very unlikely to damage yourself, which is not true of many sports. This book is about hope, my hope is that this chapter encourages you to buy a pedometer and join the many people, including many of my patients, who swear by its benefits and have biomedical tests to prove that what they feel is happening to them is a reality.

Now for the ultimate combination—one can put together walking and chanting and feel truly brilliant. A further proof of this came to me recently. I had been sent back to the cardiologist because of high blood pressure, notwithstanding the tablets I was already taking. The fascinating thing was he put me on the treadmill and the faster I went the lower my blood pressure became. It's funny because I know I feel really good when walking/chanting silently—all tension dissipates. I now understand why high blood pressure gets called hyper tension!

In the previous chapter, I have talked about chant. Normally chant is learned by sitting in the prescribed position with head tilted forwards, chin close to the chest. When one learns the technique originally, I think this is required. However, once mastered, chant can be combined with walking. If done this way you will find your long-distance ability rises greatly. Sore joints and muscles afflict one less and there is a high feel good factor.

Yes, I'm sure you have guessed it; what better way to put the whole thing together—take a walk in the country, get chanting and, if you are by the sea, a river or a lake, have a swim. You will feel amazing. My son, Cameron, and I were walking a couple of years ago in the Lake District. He can walk and swim but he doesn't chant, nor did he realise that I did. It's important to say if you get into it, it's not noticeable to others—you do not look like a nutter. We had decided to go to Coniston, walk a few miles down the lake and then climb by the back route up The Old Man of Coniston and then return from the summit by the front steep route which handily comes out at a great pub, The Sun. It's always full of climbers and hill walkers, all with a big thirst to slake. We kicked off in the early morning, designed to prevent our mistake of the previous year where we ran out of daylight and couldn't make the top. This fine day we walked most of the length of the lake, but didn't swim as we had planned, again we were in a hurry. We then headed uphill through beautiful rough countryside with a babbling brook until we reached about 2000 feet. We came around a corner to find a big lake, known as a tarn. Behind it was a huge cliff, with climbers on ropes scaling their way up, that's what I call dangerous. We sat to watch with our binoculars as a few others were doing. The next thing that happens is an English lady with her husband strips off to her bra and pants and jumps in the tarn. She is swimming around happily chatting to her husband who is sitting on the shore. I looked at Cameron: "if she can do that, so can we." We had our swimming trunks with us and quickly changed. In we went; we were squealing like pigs, wow was it cold. We have a family rule, three strokes out, three back and head under qualifies as a swim, just! I think we managed five strokes each way. The charming English lady shouted over "you are a pair of Scottish wimps" and we had to agree. We got out with cold muscles and then hit the steepest part of the climb. Age before beauty, it was time for Cameron to carry the rucksack. We arrived at the top of this hill and then took a traverse with a very nasty drop off to the left. I said to Cameron, "eyes on the narrow path, not the drop, my boy."

We arrived at the summit where much weed was being smoked, not by us. We then began our descent and by a remarkable stroke of luck got chatting to an English couple. She was an occupational health therapist and her boyfriend worked at the salt factory that lies south of the Lakes. They were good people. Suddenly, at a narrow bit, I lost my footing and spun round, only my alpine pole saving me from going straight over the edge of the cliff. I even saw the mountain rescue people were sitting at the bottom below us. I, having saved myself, then spun round and saved myself going the other way again with my Alpine pole, but to my horror this spun back to the original precipice; the woman caught my arm and saved me. Wow was I glad to have met this couple, beers on me at The Sun later, that was for sure. When we dropped down the rescue people said to me, "That was you, wasn't it, that almost fell off?" It was. I had been lucky, others not so, looking at all the grave markers in that area. I told the story to a climbing friend, who recalled that when he had been at school climbing in that area on a school trip, one of the boy's webbing strap on those old-fashioned ruck sacs had broken at a similar point, the bag coming loose and swinging the poor guy to his death. Much beer was drunk in the Sun pub that evening. This story is perhaps not the best example of combining walking, chanting and swimming, I may not be selling it well, but it was certainly memorable.

Walk the walk, swim the swim, chant the chant and maybe put them all together.

Rule 12.

Fertility, sex and orgasms are life essentials

Fertility as part of being Cup Half full

Fertility, for those who manage to preserve it through their cancer diagnosis and treatment, proves a very powerful stimulus to being cup half full. This all comes back to the holistic approach to a patient who is cared for in mind, body and spirit.

It is an interesting thought that, although the four cusps were designed for cancer patients, a three Cusp model also applies to the infertility patient. With modern management, the majority of women will have a baby, in other words they will be cured of their infertility, but many will spend long periods of uncertainty living with their infertility before they either achieve their goal or not.

A	B	C
Short term infertility	living with infertility	unable to have a baby

To give you some statistics around trying for a baby which may surprise you; if you have 100 women trying, six months after they start, fifty of them are pregnant, in other words 6 months is the average time to fall pregnant. At twelve months after trying, eighty are pregnant. This equates to 15% per month. Not what people think when they have probably spent many years making sure they don't become pregnant. Of the twenty who are left, half of them will be pregnant at 24 months out. The remaining ten will need treatment but eight or nine of them will achieve this with modern management. A diagnosis of infertility is made when a couple have tried for a baby for twelve months without success. It is also note-worthy that the data shows it is better not to try timing of sexual intercourse around ovulation but rather just to have regular inter-course throughout the month, two to four times per week, to make sure there will always be sperms around whenever the egg appears!

The other interesting set of statistics relate to age and fertil-ity. This can often be misunderstood. If you take three groups of women who are infertile and are in an IVF programme, one is 28 years of age, one 38, and the other 42, what are the chances of success? The 28-year-old has a greater than 50% chance of success at first treatment and if she were to have six cycles of IVF will get close to 90% success. Remember that those trying naturally usu-ally need six cycles. I heard an piece on BBC Radio Four not so long ago where the success of IVF was quoted at 30% and this was described as poor, but this is twice natural conception rates in a fertile couple! The 30% in fact applies to the 38-year-old woman at first treatment, with six treatments she will get to almost 80%

success. Contrast this with the 42-year-old who has a 5% chance of success at first treatment rising to 25% after 6 cycles. The great watershed is therefore at forty. For the woman who is 45 years plus she has a 1% chance per year of achieving pregnancy and by the age of 50 years a woman who gets pregnant has a 50% chance of having a hydatidiform mole, a form of cancer of the placenta often requiring chemotherapy.

These facts are important when discussing fertility issues with all patients, particularly those who have cancer and may be contemplating treatments with lesser cure rates—realism is required above plain hope. Having said this the analogy with cancer cure rates also applies, namely statistics apply to populations not individuals.

Another interesting and important fact when counselling women about their possible surgical options is the data around menopause. We talked about this earlier in respect of standard distribution curves. The average age is 51 but there are four ways of trying to guess when this might happen for a woman. What age a woman's mother went through the menopause often is helpful, estimation by blood tests of anti-Mullerian hormone (AMH) and blood tests done on the second to fifth day of the period for follicle stimulating hormone (FSH) and Oestradiol, coupled with an ultrasound estimating antral follicle count and ovarian volume. All of these factors need to be taken into account when counselling a woman about her treatment options. These factors around the female biological clock are of ever increasing importance as women are generally choosing to start families later, for various and complex reasons, thus fuelling the drive to store eggs and embryos.

Egg freezing is much in the press and happily has become more successful. To do this a woman has to go through drug-induced ovarian stimulation cycles to allow eggs to be collected and snap frozen. The success runs at 2 - 3 % per egg and therefore if twenty eggs are retrieved a 40 - 60 % chance of the desired result. Embryo freezing is much more successful, above 80% but if a woman does this with a known partner he has joint ownership. If she uses an anonymous sperm donor the woman owns the embryo, but of course they may prove to be unwanted if she then meets a partner three years later and he wants an embryo with his own sperm.

The combination of a cancer diagnosis combined with fertility issues is of course a devastating combination. It usually arises in the context that the cancer treatment will harm fertility. If a woman is going to have pelvic radiotherapy this will destroy her eggs, if she is going to have chemotherapy for any cancer, not just those gynaecological, this therapy will probably knock five to ten years off her reproductive life. All the statistics used above have to be adjusted to take this into account. If she loses her uterus, adoption and surrogacy are currently her only option, although as you saw in the first chapter that is hopefully about to change. In addition, some women are diagnosed with their cancer as part of their fertility investigations. These big issues all come crowding in at the time of initial diagnosis; this is a very hard place to find one's self.

When it comes to sexual function and orgasm this is a difficult subject to discuss with the woman about possibly to undergo a hysterectomy, but it is important that the issue is addressed. Most of the literature on this shows that, contrary to modern popular belief, a woman's sexual function either remains the same or is in fact enhanced by hysterectomy. This is not as surprising as one might think if one considers that these uteruses being removed are in fact diseased and may be causing symptoms, e.g. bleeding, pain during sex, bleeding after sex etc. However, what there is much less literature about is orgasmic function. To be slightly facile, there are probably four types of women in this respect: women who achieve orgasms from external stimulation, the majority; those that achieve it from deep internal stimulation; those that achieve it from neither and those that achieve it from both. Of those who have orgasms from deep internal stimulation, the majority likely do this via the anterior vaginal wall about two thirds of the way up, the famous and much disputed G Spot, not much disputed it has to be said by those that have one! However, there are a small proportion of women who get deep orgasms from the cervix. I use exactly the phraseology above when counselling patients and about 10% when I talk about the cervix will spontaneously say, "That's me." This small group may have their sex lives spoiled by total hysterectomy which involves removal of the cervix and body of the uterus. Sometimes it is possible to offer a subtotal hysterectomy with preservation of the cervix. Over the years I have certainly performed subtotal hysterectomies against all the guidelines in pursuit of the understandable woman's desire for maintenance of sexual function. In one woman with a cancer in the body of her uterus but not in the cervix, I cored out the cervix from the inside and she told me later that all was still in working order; this patient had told me she would refuse all surgery and die if I would not let her keep her cervix. Over the years a few women have refused the surgery after this counselling, not where they had a cancer but were at high risk of developing it.

Raffi Challion, an American professor of gynaecological oncology, was a medical student with me many years ago and went off to New York to do his elective with my friend Giuseppe Del Priore. We had set him up with a project to survey members of the British Gynaecological Cancer Society (BGCS) and New York gynaecologists as to their views on total versus subtotal hysterectomy. This made for some interesting results. The statistically significant findings being that you were less likely to be offered a subtotal hysterectomy the older your surgeon was. You were more likely to be offered a total hysterectomy if he/she was a non-oncological or benign surgeon rather than a cancer surgeon and it made no difference if your surgeon was a man or a woman. The reason given by the benign surgeons for removal of the cervix was to prevent cervical cancer. Of course, if a woman retains her cervix she must keep having cervical smears, if the cervix is removed these are usually not required. Raffi memorably presented this work at a big American meeting. Before the days of PowerPoint presentation, we used to use slides and if you were going to a big meeting it was vital that you had your slides mounted between two sheets of glass, not plastic! This was known as glassing your slides.

I had the electrifying experience of giving a talk at a World AIDS conference in Berlin to an audience of over 2000 people. At these huge meetings, you always had to remember the slide projection screen was like the screen at the Odeon, Leicester Square—massive. The projectors had enormously strong and hot light bulbs. There were four of us speaking in the session and we were all terrified. The first speaker got to the podium, asked for his first slide and it melted in an instant, same with the second slide, by the third he had to give up and slink off the podium. Of course, the other three of us were now in a worse state, had we glassed or not? We had.

On this day with Raffi he hadn't, but it was a smaller audience and his slides turned brown at 30 seconds and disappeared at 60 seconds. This guaranteed his talk ran to time and he coped very well. This work was published and we then followed with a survey of the female staff of the Chelsea and Westminster hospital. We told the staff in a letter the facts outlined above as to orgasmic habit and then asked them which operation they would choose. The significant finding was that the medical and nursing staff elected for subtotal and the ancillary and clerical staff for total hysterectomy. We submitted this work to a British journal and got the worst review of any paper I have ever seen or been involved with, the work being described as utter rubbish. Satisfyingly, the paper was published in a US journal soon thereafter.

It's important to always take a sexual history and the method for doing this is completely formulaic. The questions go thus: When was the first day of last your menstrual period? Are your periods regular or irregular? For how many days do you bleed? How long is your cycle or what is the minimum and maximum number of days between your periods? Do you get bleeding between your periods? Do you get pain during sex? Do you get bleeding after sex? If so to either of the latter, what is the bleeding like? When did you last have sex? Is your partner well? This set of questions are to my mind mandatory. The next question: Was that a regular partner or casual partner? This needs to be approached with more caution and the final question. When did you last have sex with somebody other than your current regular partner? This requires even more caution. This is the standard history in the STI clinic but in gynaecology clinics can sometimes be misinterpreted, as you will see.

I was sitting in my clinic in Charing Cross many years ago and that morning had a doctor from Greece as my observer. He had come over to do research with me over a three year period. A few weeks into his new job he had started coming to clinic as an observer and, on this particular morning between patients, he had asked me if he could start to see patients. I had said yes, but he would need to sort himself out with a defence union—there were three of these organisations at that time providing indemnity in case of one being sued. I gave him the name of two possible companies who might indemnify him and dispatched him from clinic to go make some calls and find out prices.

Meanwhile Geraldine, our staff nurse, showed in the next patient. She was an attractive woman and very vivacious. I started to take my history and ran through the questions as outlined above.

When I asked her "When did you last have sex?" She smiled and said "Four days ago in Tenerife." The venue is not part of sexual history taking, I may say. I then say "Was that your regular partner or a casual partner?" She replies "Oh you are very naughty doctor." I clock that this isn't going quite as planned but say "No, it's just a straight up question, was he a boyfriend you met there or took with you?" Not a clever phraseology on my part. She responds "Ooh, he was my regular English boyfriend." I decide to cut and run. I ask her to go behind the curtains and take her clothes off so I could examine her. The staff nurse goes with her, the curtains are pulled. Unbeknownst to patient and nurse my observer walks back into the room. I look up and ask him, "How much is it then?" before he could reply, from behind the curtains comes the reply from the patient instead "Oh I'm not a working girl, doctor, but I have a friend who could help you." Talk about giving the wrong impression!

Fertility, sex and orgasms are life essentials—that was our golden rule here, so important for almost everybody and vital to good patient care that these issues are addressed; it does not, however, always run smoothly.

Conclusion

I can't help but quote Dr Samuel Johnson "What is written without effort, is in general read without pleasure." I can promise you I've put the effort in. I can only hope that you have derived some pleasure. All of us are touched by cancer in some way, be it ourselves, our family members or our friends. Ten percent of the population have fertility problems and a few unfortunate people have the two issues intertwined. The point of this book has been to argue for the genuine empowerment of those women and their relatives who have these problems. Information is power and correct information only comes via the truth being told by all. Cancer and infertility are societally difficult to discuss, they frighten people; a lot of this book is on the edge of social acceptability, but these are the issues which do need to be brought out into the open. This allows empowerment and that leads to hope.

Different people respond in radically different ways to the same news. The other goal of the book is to show that there are many ways to discover how to live in the moment of now, one just needs to grasp them. Living in the moment of now, not thinking about the past and not worrying about the future requires work for all of us, but it is imminently possible if you have the right toolbox; the one that suits you. I venture to hope I may have made you laugh a bit too along the way. I started the book stating that it was about hope, hope of a cure, hope of living and dying well with a bad diagnosis, hope of having a baby. If this proves impossible there is the hope of good strategies to live well with the issues this creates.

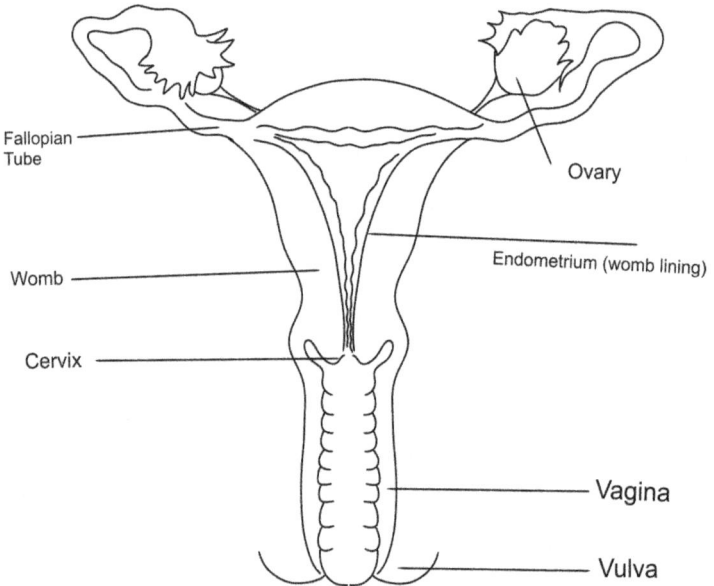

Fig 13: Anatomic picture of the female genital tract

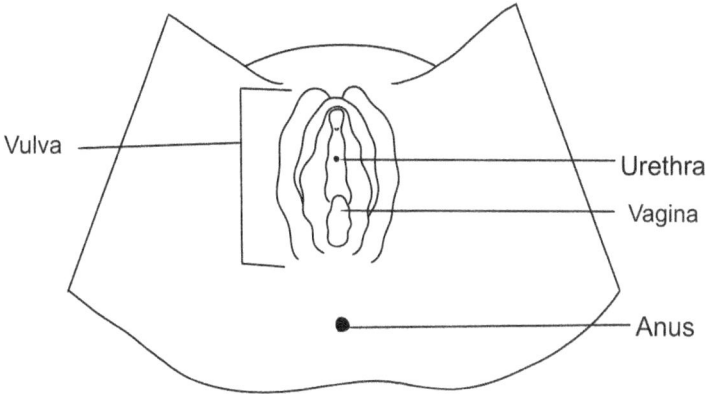

Vulva

Urethra

Vagina

Anus

Fig 14: Anatomic picture of the female external genitals

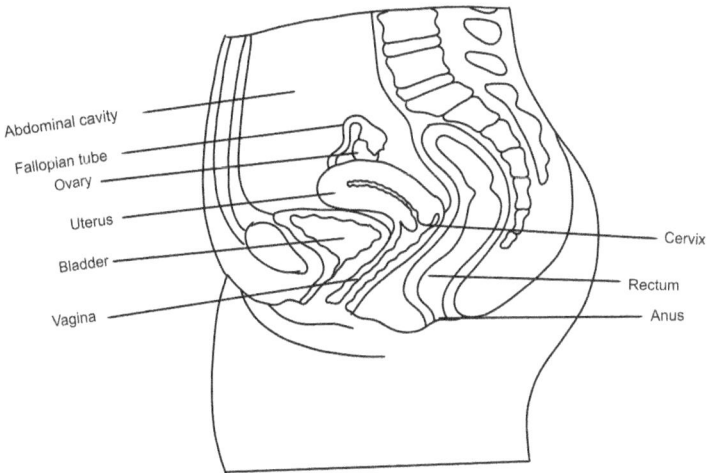

Abdominal cavity

Fallopian tube

Ovary

Uterus

Bladder

Vagina

Cervix

Rectum

Anus

Acknowledgements

To John Harrison, who was prepared to represent this book written for the public, and to support the long and special process of its incarnation. Catrina Donegan, who has spent much time covering for me in the care of my children, thus allowing this and many another project to come to light. My thanks also to my sister, Alison Smith, who has helped with many books and other projects. Also, many thanks to Syma Debbane who much encouraged and influenced the writing of this book.

Also to the late Roger Houghton, Nina Martin-Brown and the late Ann Martin, literary agents without whose teaching, guidance and encouragement this book and all my books for the public would never have been produced.

My thanks also go to Mr Sam Abdalla, Mr Shaun Hammond, Dr Tony Yardley-Jones, and the Rev. Gary Bradley, all of whom, over time, have shaped much of the thinking in this book. I would also like to thank Ms Rodena Kelman and Mrs Sue Meara for all their secretarial support, without which there would be no books. My thanks go to Mr Benjamin Jones for reading the final copy and to him, Mr Srdjan Saso and Miss Isabel Quiroga for their support and friendship over many years pushing Womb Transplant UK forwards. The anatomic pictures are Dee MacLean's, my thanks to her and Sarah Redstone of Health Press for allowing their use. My thanks also go again to Catherine Gillespie, Chief Nurse of the State of Qatar, and Dr Mark Bower for their help with developing the 4-cusp concept. My old friend, Giuseppe Del Priore, coined the term 'fertility preservation and restoration.' My thanks also to Kostas and Petroula Stergiou, proprietors of the Petra Hotel, Patmos, and their son Christos. Their hospitality and wonderful hotel provided the environment to allow me to create the first and third drafts of this book. The second draft was written in Villa Agnandio in Kioni, Ithaki, Greece and I must warmly thank Yiorgos Moraiti, Tassos Koutsouvelis and his wife Christina Moraiti for their kindness, hospitality and printing facilities, the latter truly saving the day. I am of an age where I write on the computer and have done since the early eighties but I cannot edit on anything other than paper. I would also like to thank the Bedford family—Sara, Laurence and Henry—they have become friends through many Ithaca holidays and rendered me much assistance with this and another book.

Finally, last but by no means least, is thank you to all the patients I have had the privilege to look after through tumultuous times in their lives.

About the author

The author of this book is James Richard Smith, but he is called Richard, by those who know and like him. This follows a long family tradition of the men all having James as a first name and then being called by their middle name, this being derived from their mother's maiden name. He was born in Falkirk in Scotland, educated at Dollar Academy and thereafter Glasgow University, where he qualified with a medical degree in 1982. After this he undertook a thesis on the interaction of viruses and cervical cancer graduating with an MD from Glasgow University. He has been a Fellow of the Royal College of Obstetricians and Gynaecologists and for the last thirty years, living and working in London with the exception of a brief sabbatical in New York. He currently works as a Consultant Gynaecological Surgeon at Imperial College, London, based at Hammersmith, Queen Charlotte's and Charing Cross Hospitals. He also held a Visiting and subsequently Adjunct Associate Professorship at New York University School of Medicine from 1995 -2020. In addition, he is a Professor of Practice at Imperial College, and Honorary Consultant in Transplantation Surgery at the University of Oxford.

His current professional interests are in cancer survivorship and fertility-sparing surgery for women with cancer, and the possibilities of fertility restoration for women who have been born without a womb or had a hysterectomy, via womb transplantation. He is the Chairman of Womb Transplant UK, a charity whose goal is to fund the UK's first ten womb transplants and further research in this field. He also has a keen interest in strategies to help the cancer survivor live their life with joy, not fear, more recently leading retreats to share knowledge and help people to live in the moment of now. He has four grown up children and lives between London and an island off the west coast of Scotland.

Other books by Author

Smith, JR. *A Very Byzantine Journey*. Sacristy Press, Durham 2022

Smith JR. *The Journey: Spirituality, Pilgrimage, Chant*. Darton Longman and Todd, London 2016.

Smith JR, DelPriore G, *Women's Cancers: Pathways to Living*. World Scientific, London 2016.

Shahabi S, Smith JR, DelPriore G, *Fast Facts: Gynecological Oncology, Edition 2*, 2012.

Smith JR, DelPriore G, *Women's Cancers: Pathways to Healing*, Springer, 2009.

Smith JR, DelPriore G, Curtin J, Monaghan J, *An Atlas of Gynecologic Oncology, First Edition*, Martin Dunitz 2001.

Smith JR, DelPriore G, Curtin J, Monaghan J, *An Atlas of Gynecologic Oncology, Second Edition*, Taylor and Francis 2007.

Smith JR, DelPriore, Coleman, R, Monaghan J, *An Atlas of Gynecologic Oncology, Third Edition*, Informa 2012.

Smith JR, DelPriore G, Coleman R, Monaghan J, *An Atlas of Gynecologic Oncology, Fourth Edition*, Informa 2018.

Smith JR, Del Priore G, Saso S, Coleman R, Monaghan J, *An Atlas of Gynecologic Oncology, Fifth Edition*, Informa—commissioned for 2024.

Smith JR, DelPriore G, Healy J, *An Atlas of Gynecological Cancer Staging*, Springer 2008.

Smith JR, Baron B, *Fast Facts: HIV in Obstetrics and Gynaecology*, Health Press 1998.

Smith JR, Baron B, *Fast Facts: Gynecological Oncology Edition 1*, Health Press 1998.

Smith JR, Series Editor, *Patient Pictures*, Health Press, 14 books designed to explain procedures for patients—this series sold over 200,000 copies between 1995 and 2006.

Smith JR, Series Editor, Guide to Surgery Series. Maxwell Publishing. 5 books between 1991 and 1994 designed to explain procedures for patients.

Smith JR, Kitchen VS, *Infection in Gynaecology: Churchill Livingstone*, 1993.

Glossary of Terms

APSN: atypical placental site nodule

ART: abdominal radical trachelectomy

AUFI: absolute uterine factor infertility

Cervix: neck of the womb

CIN: cervical intraepithelial neoplasia

"ectomy": removal of an organ e.g. Appendicectomy

Epithelioid trophoblastic tumour: ETT

Endometrium: lining of the womb

Fallopian tube: the "tube" between the uterus and ovary

FIGO: Federation International Gynaecologie Oncologie, an international Committee which advise on 'staging' of disease—see below

GTD: gestational trophoblastic disease, these are tumours of the placenta including partial mole, complete hydatidiform mole, invasive mole, chorio carcinoma, placental site tumours (PSTT) and epithelioid trophoblastic tumour (ETT), also including atypical placental site nodules (APSN).

HPV: human papilloma virus

Lymph nodes: glands which are situated alongside blood vessels

Metastasis (plural = metastases): cancer which has spread from its primary (original) site, also known as secondary cancer

Omentum: fatty structure hanging from the large bowel

"oscopy": to look into an organ e.g. hysteroscopy, to look into the uterus

"ostomy": to fashion a hole in an organ e.g. colostomy: to fashion a hole in the colon (large bowel)

Ovaries: the organs which produce eggs. When they stop working is when the menopause arrives

Parametrium: tissue lying lateral to the cervix

PSTT: placental site trophoblastic tumour

Stage: The amount which a cancer has spread. Always I, II, III or IV, I being earliest, i.e. not spread and IV latest i.e. spread widely

Primary cancer: the place where the cancer has started

Secondary cancer: cancer which has spread from its original, primary site, also known as metastases

SIL: squamous intraepithelial lesion, the American equivalent word for CIN

Uterus: womb

Vagina: tube of muscular tissue and mucosa between the vulva and the cervix

VAIN: vaginal intra epithelial neoplasia—a pre-cancerous condition of of the vaginal skin

VIN: Vulval intra epithelial neoplasia—a pre-cancerous condition of the vulva

Vulva: the skin on the outside of the vagina, encompassing the labia majora (hair bearing skin), the labia minora (the inner lips) and the clitoris